M. Preiss ■ M. Grapow ■ P. Buser ■ H.-R. Zerkowski ■ (Eds.)

Cardiac Disease in the Elderly

M. Preiss   M. Grapow
P. Buser   H.-R. Zerkowski   (Eds.)

Cardiac Disease in the Elderly

Interventions
Ethics
Economics

Introduction by Carlo Conti
With 22 Figures and 21 Tables

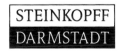

STEINKOPFF
DARMSTADT

Dr. MICHAEL PREISS   Dr. MARTIN GRAPOW
Prof. Dr. P. BUSER   Prof. Dr. HANS-REINHARD ZERKOWSKI
Universitätsklinik für Herz- und Thoraxchirurgie
Kantonsspital Basel
Spitalstraße 21, CH-4031 Basel

ISBN 3-7985-1286-8 Steinkopff Verlag Darmstadt

Die Deutsche Bibliothek – CIP-Einheitsaufnahme
A catalogue record for this publication is available from Die Deutsche Bibliothek

Steinkopff Verlag Darmstadt
a member of BertelsmannSpringer Science+Business Media GmbH

© Steinkopff Verlag Darmstadt 2001
   Printed in Germany

Medical Editor: Sabine Ibkendanz
Production: Klemens Schwind
Cover Design: Erich Kirchner, Heidelberg
Typesetting: K + V Fotosatz GmbH, Beerfelden

SPIN 10792798   85/7231-5 4 3 2 1 0 – Printed on acid-free paper

Introduction

Carlo Conti

You are today confronting sensitive questions on the subject of "Cardiac surgery and heart diseases in old age" and I congratulate you on this. It is a brave and important step to discuss this multifaceted question which demands an answer and an explanation from many perspectives:

- From a *medical* perspective, there is the question of the medical feasibility and durability of treatment.
- From an *economic* angle we ask ourselves whether we can pay for everything that is medically feasible.
- From the *patient's* perspective there is the legitimate desire and the justified need not to leave anything untried that might serve to sustain or improve the quality of life.
- The *ethical* perspective: is what is feasible really desirable? Should everything be done simply because it can be done? Is it ethically acceptable to set an age limit on an operation that in all probability will produce an improvement in the quality of life? And if so, where does this limit lie? Below it surgery is "worthwhile" but above it is not? No-one in all seriousness and with a clean conscience will want to draw this line randomly or arbitrarily. That appears to us – quite rightly – morally unacceptable.
- The *doctors'* perspective: they are obliged by the Hippocratic oath in principle to carry out all the treatments that are indicated and comply with the rules of the art of medicine.

Today, because rationing in the health system is on everyone's lips and a cost explosion is imminent, the economic perspective will also play an important role in your discussions. In the question of *rationalisation* versus *rationing* and the *affordability* of the healthcare system, patients, the medical profession, policy and the public are faced with a challenge. None of us can avoid these questions. What do we want to, and what can we, afford; who pays and who receives the service? One might also ask: where can we make savings so that we can pay for other things?

Do we still have a couple of years before everything that is technically and medically feasible bursts the bounds of the jointly financed health system?

A hospital also finances itself through medical services, through the employment of technical and staff resources, but never covers its costs. We all know that. We know from experience that what is on offer is taken up. "A built bed is a filled bed", said Milton Roemer in 1959, and this can also be applied to your subject.

My predecessor in office once said: "Health policy is the constant attempt to square the circle, in other words to finance almost unlimited medical progress for everyone with limited means," with which I agree. We all have two hearts in our chest: When we are ill, we should like to receive the best treatment and be cared for devotedly. And yet we complain of the constantly increasing health costs which place an ever greater burden on our budget. What can we do to ensure that the gap between the available resources and on-going costs does not open still wider? What is feasible and what is desirable? When is less more? Who decides? The service provider, the recipient, the politician?

Politicians who have perhaps not yet reached the age of fifty are supposed to decide what a seventy or eighty year-old needs, what care they require. Will I, in twenty or thirty years' time, find someone who will operate on me?

It is encouraging and welcome that you should take up and discuss this delicate and constantly changing topic from a wide variety of perspectives in an interdisciplinary and joint approach. I would like the discussion that you are instituting here to be continued publicly, its threads teased out further in the outside world. I welcome you here on behalf of the government and wish you a fruitful, stimulating and productive day.

Geleitwort

Carlo Conti

Sie befassen sich heute mit sensiblen Fragestellungen zum Thema „Herzchirurgie und Herzkrankheiten im Alter". Dazu beglückwünsche ich Sie. Es ist mutig und wichtig, dieses Thema zu diskutieren, diese vielschichtige Frage, die in mehreren Aspekten nach einer Beantwortung und Klärung ruft:

- Aus *medizinischer* Sicht ergibt sich die Frage nach der medizinischen Machbarkeit und nach der Nachhaltigkeit der Behandlung.
- Aus *ökonomischer* Sicht fragen wir uns, ob wir alles bezahlen können, was medizinisch machbar wäre.
- Aus der Sicht *des Patienten, der Patientin* ergibt sich der legitime Wunsch und das berechtigte Bedürfnis, nichts unversucht zu lassen, was der Erhaltung oder Verbesserung der Lebensqualität dient.
- Die *ethische* Sicht: Ist wirklich wünschenswert, was machbar ist? Soll alles durchgeführt werden, nur weil es durchführbar ist? Ist es ethisch vertretbar, für einen Eingriff, der mit der größten Wahrscheinlichkeit eine Verbesserung der Lebensqualität nach sich ziehen wird, eine Altersgrenze festzulegen? Und wenn ja, wo liegt diese? Bis hierhin „lohnt" sich eine Operation, von da an nicht mehr? Niemand wird ernsthaft und mit reinem Gewissen diese Grenze zufällig oder willkürlich ziehen wollen. Dies scheint uns – natürlich zu Recht – moralisch nicht statthaft.
- Die Sicht *der Ärztin, des Arztes*: Sie sind dem Hippokratischen Eid verpflichtet, grundsätzlich all diejenigen Therapien durchzuführen, die indiziert sind und den Regeln der medizinischen Kunst entsprechen.

Heute, da die Rationierung im Gesundheitswesen in aller Munde ist, die Kostenexplosion bedrängt, wird auch bei der

Diskussion Ihres Themas die ökonomische Sicht eine wichtige Rolle spielen. Bei der Frage *Rationalisierung* versus *Rationierung* und *Finanzierbarkeit* des Gesundheitswesens sind Patienten und Patientinnen, Ärzteschaft, Politik und Öffentlichkeit gefordert. Wir alle können uns diesen Fragen nicht entziehen. Was wollen und können wir uns leisten, wer bezahlt, wer empfängt die Leistung? Man könnte auch fragen: Wo können wir einsparen, damit anderes bezahlt werden kann?

Haben wir noch ein paar Jahre Zeit, bis alles was technisch und medizinisch machbar ist, die Grenzen des solidarisch finanzierten Gesundheitssystems sprengt?

Ein Spital finanziert sich auch durch die medizinischen Leistungen, durch die Beanspruchung der technischen und personellen Ressourcen, arbeitet aber nie kostendeckend. Das ist uns allen bekannt. Angebote, die bereitstehen, werden erfahrungsgemäß auch genutzt. „A built bed is a filled bed", sagte Milton Roemer 1959, dies lässt sich auch auf Ihr Thema übertragen.

Meine Vorgängerin im Amt hat einmal gesagt: „Gesundheitspolitik ist der ständige Versuch der Quadratur des Kreises, nämlich mit beschränkten Mitteln einen nahezu unbeschränkten medizinischen Fortschritt für alle zu finanzieren". Dem stimme ich zu. Wir alle haben zwei Herzen in unserer Brust: Wir möchten, wenn wir krank sind, optimal behandelt und hingebungsvoll gepflegt werden. Trotzdem beklagen wir uns über die ständig steigenden Gesundheitskosten, die unser Budget immer stärker belasten.

Was können wir tun, damit sich die Schere zwischen den verfügbaren Mitteln und den laufenden Kosten nicht noch weiter öffnet? Was ist machbar, was wünschenswert? Wann ist weniger mehr? Wer entscheidet? Der Leistungserbringer, die Leistungsempfängerin, der oder die Politiker?

Politiker, die vielleicht die fünfzig Jahre noch nicht erreicht haben, sollen darüber entscheiden, was ein Siebzigjähriger, eine Achtzigjährige braucht, welcher Pflege sie bedürfen. Finde ich in zwanzig, in dreißig Jahren einen, der mich operiert?

Es ist erfreulich und begrüßenswert, dass Sie aus den verschiedensten Blickwinkeln dieses heikle, bewegende Thema interdisziplinär und gemeinsam aufnehmen und diskutieren. Ich wünschte mir, die Diskussion, die Sie hier beginnen, würde öffentlich weitergeführt, der Faden draußen weitergesponnen. Ich begrüße Sie hier im Namen der Regierung und wünsche Ihnen einen fruchtbaren, anregenden, weiterführenden Tag.

Table of Contents

List of Authors

Prof. Dr. P. BUSER
Abteilung f. Kardiologie
Klinikum 2, Medizin
Petersgraben 12
4031 Basel, Schweiz

Dr. C. CONTI
Regierungsrat
Sanitätsdepartement
St.-Alban-Vorstadt 25
4051 Basel, Schweiz

Prof. Dr. R. S. HARTZ
Tulane University School
of Medicine
1430 Tulane Avenue
New Orleans, LA 70112, USA

Prof. Dr. M. HEBERER
Dept. Chirurgie
Kantonsspital
4031 Basel, Schweiz

A. RYCHEN
VISANA
Weltpoststr. 17–21
3000 Bern 15, Schweiz

Prof. Dr. H.-P. SCHREIBER
ETH-Zentrum
Ethik+Technologiefolgen-
Abschätzung
Rämistr. 101
8092 Zürich, Schweiz

Prof. Dr. H. B. STAEHELIN
Universitätsklinik f. Geriatrie
Kantonsspital
Spitalstr. 21
4031 Basel, Schweiz

Prof. Dr. M. WEHR
Klinik f. Kardiologie u. Angiologie
Augusta-Krankenanstalt
Bergstr. 26
44791 Bochum

G. ZISSELSBERGER
AOK-Gesundheitskasse Lörrach
Bezirksdirektion der AOK BW
Weilerstr. 19–21
79540 Lörrach

Prof. Dr. P. ZWEIFEL
Socioeconomic Institute
Hottingerstr. 10
8032 Zürich, Schweiz

CHAPTER **1** **Cardiac disease in the elderly –**
the true millennium problem

H. B. STAEHELIN

■ Introduction

The 20th century experienced a dramatic increase in life expectancy. This change was driven by two factors, namely the massive decline in infant mortality, mortality throughout adolescence and young adulthood, and secondly by a substantial increase of life expectancy which for the great majority in industrialized societies has resulted in a third age period (65–75), and for an increasing number a fourth age period (75+). The successful treatment of infectious disease, improvement in nutrition, hygiene, lifestyle and living conditions now allows a life expectancy at birth for Switzerland of 81.6 years for women and 76.4 years for men [7]. Life expectancy for persons at 65 has doubled over the last 100 years from 10 to 16.7 years for men and from 6.5 to 20 years for women. Mortality due to infectious diseases has shifted to mortality due to chronic degenerative diseases and neoplastic diseases. However, during the second half of the 20th century, premature death (defined as death before 65) declined dramatically, mostly thanks to a sharp reduction in cardiovascular death. However, data demonstrate the exponential increase in cardiovascular mortality from age 65 to 85+ for men and women [10], whereas the cancer mortality increases more linearly [6]. Data from Switzerland give the same results [7]. In the older population we observe a decline in the age-adjusted cardiovascular mortality but compared to the below 65 year olds to a lesser extent. Over the same time span, death due to neoplastic disease remained constant or increased slightly. A comparison between industrialized culture with distinctly different nutritional habits and life styles (e.g., Japan and the UK) demonstrate similar patterns.

■ Conceptual framework of the longevity revolution

The longevity we experience at present exposes the aging individual to increased vulnerability. There is good evidence that biological evolution has been optimized by natural selection up to the age of about 50. Benefits resulting from evolutionary selection decrease with progressing age [5], and we observe-among other factors an increasingly larger number of dysfunctional gene expressions, an accumulation of dysfunctional proteins, and impaired repair functions (Fig. 1). Selection operating through reproduction has thus a small effect in the second half of life. In order to continue life successfully, cultural influences become increasingly prominent. Nevertheless, with age and external conditions contributing to the primarily negative biological development of the life course, the relative effectiveness of external psychological and social interventions diminish. Much effort has to be made to maintain function and to compensate for losses. One may conceptualize, according to Baltes, this development as *selective optimization with compensation* [1]. From these theoretical considerations it may easily be deduced that medical care becomes increasingly important with advancing age.

■ Impact on heart disease

The reduction in incidence of heart disease leads only partly to an overall reduction in cardiovascular morbidity and mortality. It shifts mortality from the third to the fourth age period.

The age-adjusted presentation of the data in the past misled to the thinking that cardiovascular morbidity and mortality are less impor-

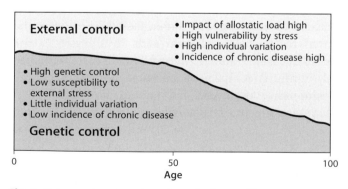

Fig. 1. Nature and nurture throughout the human life span

Table 1. Causes of death in persons aged 75 and over

Cause of death	Men [%]	Women [%]
Cardiovascular	48	55
Cancer	30	30
Other	22	15

Table 2. Manageable risk factors for CVD

- Smoking
- Obesity
- High levels of alcohol consumption
- Unsuitable nutrition
- Lack of physical exercise
- Elevated total and low density lipoprotein [LDL] cholesterol

tant. Particularly the fact that cardiovascular disease is significantly less frequent in women below 75 compared to men of the same age group has led in the past to an underestimation of the true impact of cardiovascular disease in women (Table 1). As an overall cause of mortality, cardiovascular disease is even more prominent in women than in men.

Given the fact that an increasing number of elderly persons reach a high age, cardiovascular disease contributes enormously to the health care burden. It ranks first as cause of death and second as cause of disability [6, 10]. We note an increasing prevalence of heart failure and stroke with advancing age. Rich states in a recent review that over 75% of patients with heart failure are 65 or older [9]. It is the leading cause for hospitalization in older adults. In the Framingham Study the incidence of heart failure declined over time (per decade 11% for men and 17% for women (less than for coronary artery disease)) and shows poor survival, namely a median 5-year survival for men 25% and 38% for women [3]. Successful medical treatment, however, contributes not only to the shift of cardiac morbidity to higher ages but also to higher hospital admission and readmission rates [8].

The importance of risk factors in the development of cardiovascular disease is well established (Table 2). The recent report from the Nurses Health Study demonstrated a 31% decline in coronary heart disease over a 14 year period [4]. Less smoking contributed 13%, hormonal replacement therapy 9%, and particularly impressive was improved diet 16% (Fig. 2). Some of the advances were offset by an increasing preva-

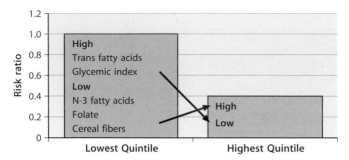

Fig. 2. Impact of diet on coronary heart disease [4]

lence (+38%) of obesity. Given the trend in obesity prevalence, we thus may anticipate a reversal of the age-adjusted decline of cardiovascular disease in the years ahead or at least an important effect on cardiovascular disease in the coming years.

Intervention trials with lipid lowering drugs and antihypertensives extending into old age demonstrate – even in the population of 75+ – treatment benefits. We thus may reduce morbidity and mortality. There is, however, still a substantial reluctance to continue adequate risk factor treatment in elderly subjects, and trials within larger populations are rare. Given the large number of older subjects at risk and the high incidence, treatment efficacy is even greater in the older than in the younger population at risk with low incidence. It is only reluctantly that aggressive lipid lowering and antihypertensive therapy is adopted, despite the well-established benefits and collateral effects on fractures and osteoporosis of statins and, to a lesser extent, thiazide diuretics.

The increasing number of older patients will pose the question of treatment goals and access to treatment. The demographic changes will undoubtedly lead to more medical and surgical interventions. The aggressive early detection of persons at risk and the treatment of risk factors remain important goals. Chronic cardiovascular disease is not only the leading cause of mortality, but also one of the leading causes of disability. Chronic heart failure severely impairs quality of life, cognitive function, and autonomy of the patient. Indeed, these functional and inactive years at the end of life become increasingly important with higher age. As shown above, men are at higher risk for heart failure and their prognosis is worse than in women. Longer life expectancy, however, does not imply longer healthy life. Men and women will experience prolonged periods of dependency in old age (Table 3). As shown in Table 3, women more so than men [2]. One reason may be the superior muscle strength of men.

Table 3. Remaining life expectancy and estimated dysfunctional years

Age	70	80	90
Women	14	8	5
Dysfunctional years	2.8	2.8	3
Men	10	6	3
Dysfunctional years	1.6	1.6	1.6

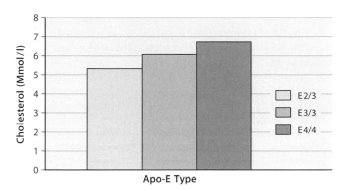

Fig. 3. Apolipoprotein E and plasma cholesterol

The fact that we are able to prevent and delay cardiovascular disease and treat it with increasing effectiveness raises new interesting aspects. It is now well established that the apolipoprotein E polymorphism is related to the susceptibility for cardiovascular disease. Thus, apolipoprotein E4 is associated with higher cholesterol level compared to apo E3 or E2 (Fig. 3). It has been shown that heterozygous apolipoprotein E4 carriers are 3–4 times more susceptible to suffer from Alzheimer's disease, homozygous carriers 8–9 times. The disease develops earlier in life and occurs more frequently. Preventing and treating the increased risk of cardiovascular morbidity and mortality in apo E4 subjects exposes them to a higher chance of experiencing Alzheimer's disease. This indicates the limits of prevention. It also explains part of the ambiguity towards medical progress in the population.

The goal of medicine in old age will be to compensate for loss of function and thus lessen disability and dependency in old age. Early detection of persons at risk, treating risk factors and optimizing cardiovascular function may contribute greatly to successful aging by diminishing chronic heart failure and cardiovascular disease.

▪ References

1. Baltes PB (1997) On the incomplete architecture of human ontogeny. Selection, optimization, and compensation as foundation of developmental theory. Am Psychol 52:366–380
2. Crimmins EM, Hayward MD, Saito Y (1996) Differentials in active life expectancy in the older population of the United States. J Gerontol B Psychol Sci Soc Sci 51:S111–S200
3. Ho DS, Cooper MJ, Richards DA et al (1993) Comparison of number of extrastimuli versus change in basic cycle length for induction of ventricular tachycardia by programmed ventricular stimulation. J Am Coll Cardiol 22:1711–1717
4. Hu FB, Stampfer MJ, Manson JE et al (2000) Trends in the incidence of coronary heart disease and changes in diet and lifestyle in women. N Engl J Med 343:530–537
5. Martin GM, Austad SN, Johnson TEJ (1996) Genetic analysis of ageing: role of oxidative damage and environmental stresses. Nat Genet 13:25–34
6. Murray CJ, Lopez AD (1997) Global mortality, disability, and the contribution of risk factors: Global Burden of Disease Study. Lancet 349:1436–1442/Murray CJ, Lopez AD (1997) Mortality by cause for eight regions of the world: Global Burden of Disease Study. Lancet 349:1269–1276
7. Pharma Information (1999) Das Gesundheitswesen in der Schweiz, Ausgabe 1999. Pharma Information, Basel
8. Reitsma JB, Mosterd A, de Craen AJ et al (1996) Increase in hospital admission rates for heart failure in The Netherlands. 76:388–392
9. Rich MW (1997) Epidemiology, pathophysiology, and etiology of congestive heart failure in older adults. J Am Geriatr Soc 45:968–974
10. World Development Report (1993) Investing in health. The International Bank for Reconstruction and Development, Washington DC

■ Herzkrankheit im Alter – Das wahre Millenium-Problem

H. B. STAEHELIN

Die eindrucksvolle Zunahme der individuellen Lebenserwartung im 20. Jahrhundert war das Resultat einer starken Reduktion der Sterblichkeit an Infektionskrankheiten im Kindes- und frühen Erwachsenenalter und einer erfolgreichen Behandlung chronischer Krankheiten im mittleren Erwachsenenalter. Der altersadjustierte Rückgang der Morbidität und Mortalität der Herzkreislaufkrankheiten darf aber nicht darüber hinweg täuschen, dass diese weiterhin die führende Todesursache darstellen und bei über 75-jährigen Frauen für 55%, bei Männern für 48% aller Todesfälle verantwortlich sind. 75% aller Patienten mit Herzinsuffizienz sind 65 Jahre oder älter. Herzinsuffizienz ist die führende Hospitalisationsursache im höheren Lebensalter. Betrachtet vor dem theoretischen Hintergrund des Konzepts der selektiven Optimierung und Kompensation und der Beobachtung, dass genetische Faktoren im dritten und vierten Lebensalter zunehmend an Einfluss verlieren, ergibt sich ein steigender Bedarf an medizinischen Leistungen zur Aufrechterhaltung der Gesundheit und Autonomie. Früh einsetzende und nachhaltige präventive Maßnahmen, die auf eine Modifikation der Risikofaktoren abzielen, haben in den vergangenen Jahren zu einem weiteren Rückgang der kardiovaskulären Morbidität und Mortalität geführt. Gleichzeitig hat aber der starke Anstieg der Prävalenz der Obesitas einen Teil dieser Verbesserung wieder zunichte gemacht. Der immer noch ansteigende Trend in der Prävalenz der Obesitas dürfte in Zukunft die Zahl der Herzkreislaufkrankheiten wieder früher auftreten und noch häufiger werden lassen. Durch die Aufklärung des Einflusses bestimmter genetischer Polymorphismen (z. B. Apolipoprotein E4) auf den Lipidstoffwechsel, aber auch auf andere chronisch degenerative Krankheiten, wird es in Zukunft möglich sein, individuell selektive Präventivstrategien zu entwickeln.

CHAPTER 2

Coronary interventions in the elderly – the German ALKK Study Group experience

M. Wehr, A. Vogt, C. Pfafferott, E. Grube,
H.-G. Glunz
(for the ALKK Study Group)

Percutaneous transluminal coronary angioplasty (PTCA) is offered only reluctantly to elderly patients, as the general conviction is that this invasive form of treatment carries a substantial risk whilst offering only modest benefits [1, 5, 6]. However, in the last few years interventional techniques have improved and stents have become more widely used, and it is especially in elderly patients that success rates have risen and complication rates fallen [3, 4]. The effectiveness of PTCA is seen in angiographic and functional results, improvements in clinical symptoms and quality of life and finally also in cost [2].

Here we report our retrospective short- and long-term results of PTCA in patients over 80 years of age from the ALKK register for 1993 (pre-stent era).

▪ Patients

One hundred and fifty-three patients with an average age of over 82 years (88 men and 65 women) who underwent PTCA in 1993 in one of the 33 ALKK centres were included in the study. Data were collected from doctors' letters. Six-year follow-up data for 110 patients were recorded by means of a questionnaire completed by the attending cardiologist or family doctor.

▪ Pre-existing conditions

Figure 1 summarises the pre-existing conditions elicited in these 153 patients.

Fifty-eight had had a previous infarct, and 39 a previous anterior wall infarct. An acute myocardial infarct was present in 24 patients (anterior wall 12, posterior wall 9, not localised 3) and 3 patients had cardiogenic shock. A total of 56 patients had three-vessel coronary dis-

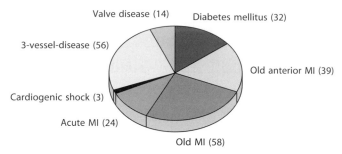

Valve disease (14)   Diabetes mellitus (32)

3-vessel-disease (56)

Old anterior MI (39)

Cardiogenic shock (3)

Acute MI (24)

Old MI (58)

Fig. 1. Baseline characteristics, 153 patients

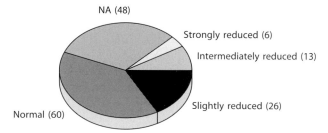

NA (48)

Strongly reduced (6)

Intermediately reduced (13)

Normal (60)

Slightly reduced (26)

Fig. 2. LV-ejection fraction, 153 patients

ease, 14 had valvular disease and 32 had diabetes mellitus. Two-thirds of the patients had anginal symptoms of CCS grade II to IV.

▪ Ejection fraction

Figure 2 shows the available left ventricular ejection fraction data for the study patients. The ejection fraction was normal or slightly reduced in 86 patients, moderately impaired in 13 and severely impaired in 6. No data were available for the remaining 48 patients.

▪ Dilated vessels

Figure 3 shows the vessels that were dilated. In 68 patients the left anterior descending artery (LAD) was dilated, in 30 the circumflex artery (RCX), in 31 the right coronary artery (RCA) and in 2 patients the left main stem. Secondary branches were dilated in 5 patients, an aortocoronary bypass vein graft was dilated in 2 patients and in 15 patients two vessels were dilated in one session.

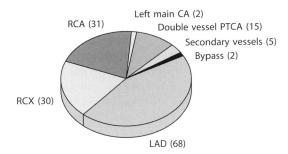

Fig. 3. Dilated vessels, 153 patients

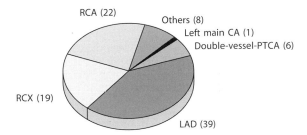

Fig. 4. 'Prima vista PTCA',
83 patients

▪ 'Prima vista' PTCA

A so-called 'prima vista' PTCA (i.e. coronary angiography and PTCA in one session) was performed in 83 patients (54.3%), 24 of whom were in the acute phase of myocardial infarction. Figure 4 shows the vessels treated (39 LAD, 19 circumflex, 22 RCA, 8 other vessels and 1 main stem). In 6 patients two vessels were dilated in one session.

▪ Results

PTCA was unsuccessful in 7 patients (4.6%) and led unavoidably to the deaths of 2 patients (1.3%). PTCA of the right coronary artery failed in an 84-year-old man with a history of anterior and posterior wall infarction and severe three-vessel coronary disease who was admitted with cardiogenic shock due to a new posterior wall infarct. An 83-year-old woman with a history of anterior and posterior wall infarction and known mitral insufficiency was admitted with unstable angina (CCS grade IV). PTCA of the circumflex artery was attempted unsuccessfully and the patient died of a further infarct.

A Q-wave infarct was noted in 13 patients (8.5%) after PTCA. Seven of these had had PTCA because of an acute myocardial infarct. Thus,

Table 1. PTCA – acute results, 153 patients

PTCA failure:	n = 7	(4.6%)
■ Death	n = 2	(1.3%)
■ Q-MI	n = 13	(AMI: n = 7)
■ TLR	n = 2	

Table 2. PTCA follow-up results (6 yrs), general living conditions

Patient alive	56
■ lives alone, no nursing care	18
■ lives with partner, no nursing care	13
■ lives without partner but with family	6
■ lives alone, receives nursing care	12
■ lives with partner, receives nursing care	1
■ lives in nursing home	5
■ NA	1

PTCA prevented a Q-wave infarct in 17 out of 24 patients with acute myocardial infarct. Surgical revascularisation was necessary in 2 patients (1.3%). These results are summarized in Table 1.

Six-year follow-up (Table 2) was possible in 110 patients (a drop-out rate of 28%).

Of these 110 patients, 56 were still alive (51%). Those who died survived an average of 39.9 months. The cause of death was cardiac in 14, non-cardiac in 13 and unknown in 14 patients.

Six years after PTCA, 37 of the 56 patients (66%) did not need nursing care – 18 lived alone, 13 with partner and 6 without a partner but with family). Nursing care was necessary in 18 of the 56 survivors (32%), of whom one lived with a partner, 12 lived alone and 5 were in nursing homes. Details were not available for one patient.

The clinical efficacy of PTCA for the 110 patients is shown in Tables 3 and 4.

Anginal symptoms improved in 75 of the 110 patients (69%). Fifty-five of the 110 (50%) reported an improvement in their general state of health and 44 (40%) said that their general living circumstances had changed for the better.

In 27 of the 110 patients (24%), cardioactive medication could be reduced and 40 patients (37%) needed no further hospital admission for cardiac treatment. Eleven patients underwent a further PTCA and 5 a

Table 3. PTCA follow-up results (6 yrs), clinical efficacy I

Angina pectoris after PTCA	
▪ less	75
▪ unchanged	3
▪ NA	32
General health status after PTCA	
▪ better	55
▪ unchanged	15
▪ worse	3
▪ NA	37
General living circumstances after PTCA	
▪ better	44
▪ unchanged	30
▪ worse	3
▪ NA	33

Table 4. PTCA follow-up results (6 yrs), clinical efficacy II

Medication before and after PTCA	
▪ more	9
▪ less	27
▪ unchanged	32
▪ NA	42
Hospitalisation after PTCA	
yes	38
▪ PTCA	11
▪ CABG	5
▪ Pacemaker implant	2
▪ Heart failure	13
no	40
NA	42

coronary artery bypass operation. Two patients received a cardiac pace-maker and 13 required in-patient treatment for heart failure.

Comparison of the PTCA results in this study with PTCA data from the ALKK register for the year 1999 – a total of 27 099 younger patients aged 63.7 ± 10.5 years – shows similar results. Therefore, PTCA repre-

Table 5. PTCA – register (1999), n = 27 099

▪ Age (yrs)	63.7 ± 10.5
▪ Females	26.1%
▪ 3-Vessel disease	26.3%
▪ AMI	8.92%
▪ PTCA infarct	0.85%
▪ Death	1.07%
▪ Death, emergency surgery or MI	1.64%

sents a significant palliative procedure even in the elderly and is not associated with excess morbidity and mortality.

The above investigation shares with all retrospective studies the problems of selection bias and missing data. Not all patients over 80 who underwent PTCA were treated in a participating centre and are, thus, missing from the register. Also, some patients from ALKK centres who underwent PTCA in 1993 were not included in the analysis.

▪ Conclusion

In selected patients advanced age is not in itself a contraindication to PTCA. This seems to apply particularly to patients with an acute myocardial infarct. PTCA is an effective therapy with an acceptable complication rate even in patients over 80 years of age and the threshold for its use can be lowered. A prospective study which includes patients from this age group is long overdue.

▪ References

1. Jackmann JD, Navetta FL, Smith JE et al. (1991) Percutaneous transluminal coronary angioplasty in octogenarians as an effective therapy for angina pectoris. Am J Cardiol 68:116–119
2. Kähler J, Lütke M, Weckmüller J et al. (1999) Coronary angioplasty in octogenarians – quality of life and costs. Eur Heart J 20:1791–1798
3. Morrison DA, Bies RD, Sacks J (1997) Coronary angioplasty for elderly patients with 'high risk' unstable angina: short-term outcomes and long-term survival. J Am Coll Cardiol 29:339–344
4. Ten Berg JM, Voors AA, Suttorp MJ, et al. (1996) Long-term results after successful percutaneous transluminal coronary angioplasty in patients over 75 years of age. Am J Cardiol 77:690–705
5. Thompson RC, Holmes DR, Grill DE et al. (1996) Changing outcome of angioplasty in the elderly. J Am Coll Cardiol 27:8–14
6. Vaitkus PT, Witmer WT et al. (1997) Cardiologists' perception of risk of coronary revascularization procedures. J Cardiol 80:339–341

▪ Koronarinterventionen im Alter – Die Deutsche ALKK-Studiengruppe

M. Wehr, A. Vogt, C. Pfafferott, E. Grube, H.-G. Glunz
(für die ALKK-Studiengruppe)

Die perkutane transluminale koronare Angioplastie (PTCA) wird älteren Patienten noch zurückhaltend angeboten, da nach allgemeiner Überzeugung diese invasive Therapieform ein hohes Risiko bei nur geringer klinischer Effizienz beinhaltet [1, 5, 6]. Durch die Verbesserung der interventionellen Techniken und die zunehmende Verwendung von Stents wurden jedoch in den letzten Jahren besonders bei älteren Patienten die Erfolgsrate erhöht und die Komplikationsrate verringert [3, 4]. Die Effektivität der PTCA wird durch das angiografische und funktionelle Ergebnis, die Verbesserung der klinischen Symptomatik und Lebensqualität und letztendlich auch durch die Kosten bestimmt [6]. Wir berichten hier retrospektiv über die Akut- und Langzeitergebnisse der PTCA bei über 80-Jährigen aus dem ALKK-Register des Jahres 1993 (Nicht-Stent-Ära). 153 Patienten im mittleren Alter von über 82 Jahren (88 Männer, 65 Frauen), die sich 1993 in 33 ALKK-Kliniken einer PTCA unterziehen mussten, wurden in die Studie eingeschlossen. Die Datenerhebung erfolgte aus den vorliegenden Arztbriefen bis hin zu den sechsjährlichen Follow-up-Daten, die bei 110 Patienten mittels eines Fragebogens durch die behandelnden Kardiologen oder Hausärzte erhoben werden konnten. Die Ergebnisse zeigen, dass bei ausgewählten Patienten offensichtlich auch ein hohes Lebensalter keine generelle Kontraindikation gegen eine PTCA darstellt. Das scheint vor allem auch Patienten mit einem akuten Myokardinfarkt zu betreffen. Die PTCA ist auch bei über 80-Jährigen eine effektive Therapie mit akzeptabler Komplikationsrate, deren Indikationsschwelle gesenkt werden kann. Der Einschluss dieser Altersgruppen in ein prospektives Studiendesign erscheint daher mehr als überfällig zu sein.

CHAPTER 3 **Coronary interventions in the elderly – the Swiss Catheter Experience**

P. BUSER

■ Introduction

In cardiac catheterisation investigations and cardiac operations, the risk of complications increases markedly with advancing age, especially in patients over 75 years [1]. This is one of the reasons why cardiac catheterisation and interventional treatment of coronary heart disease were employed with relative restraint in this age group until a few years ago. It was also one of the reasons why patients older than 70–75 years were traditionally not included in randomised studies of cardiac interventions. However, when we consider that the number of persons aged over 75 years will double in Switzerland in the course of the next 20 years [2], so that naturally the number of patients with coronary heart disease requiring treatment will increase considerably, there is an urgent need to document and analyse the risks and benefits of coronary interventions in patients in this age group.

The following is a brief overview of the differences between younger and older patients in the invasive investigation and treatment of coronary heart disease and the known data on this subject from Switzerland, and the first randomised multicentre study is presented.

■ Coronary heart disease in elderly patients

A clinical epidemiological study of the inhabitants of Rochester [3] showed that in 1982 the incidence of an acute myocardial infarction per 100 000 inhabitants was 92 per year in men aged 33–44, 372 in men aged 45–54 and 735 in men aged 65–74. The incidence was 6, 270 and 560 in the corresponding age groups in women. The results were similar to those of the Framingham study. That is, the incidence of myocardial infarction increases considerably with advancing age, it is observed less frequently in women in age groups under 65 years than in men of comparable age, but with advancing age, it is comparable in women aged over 65 years to the incidence in men of the same age. If these numbers are extrapolated to the next two decades, when those born in the baby boom years will pass the age of 65 years, an enormous rise in the numbers of elderly infarct patients must be anticipated. The treatment strategies established in the 1980s and 1990s such as thrombolysis and acute PTCA have led to a marked drop in mortality due to myocardial infarction. However, this applies particularly to age groups under 65 years, both in men and women. Nevertheless, mortality in the period 1980–1994 was reduced by about 25% in 65-84 year olds also, but a rise in mortality of 3–5% was observed in the over-85 year olds [4]. Myocardial infarction is therefore more dangerous for elderly patients and the treatment strategies employed today could even increase the risk in those over 80 years. This could also be due to the fact that elderly patients have complex vessel pathology, which increases the risks of intervention. Chaitman showed in 1981 in a group of 2000 patients with coronary heart disease in the CASS study that coronary triple-branch disease and disease affecting the main stem are commoner in those over 70 compared to younger patients [5]. The realisation that complex vessel pathology is present more frequently in elderly patients with coronary heart disease led in the 1980s to invasive investigation being regarded as rather contraindicated. However, the development of catheter technique and above all the routine use of intracoronary stents in the 1990s produced a rapid increase in the invasive investigation and interventional treatment of coronary heart disease in elderly and old patients. It was shown in several small groups of patients that the improvement in both the functional status and in the quality of life after percutaneous coronary intervention in patients over 70 is comparable with that of patients under 70 years [6]. In very old patients, revascularisation also improves survival compared to conservative medical treatment [7]. In patients with moderately severe to severe heart failure, bypass surgery appears to be superior to percutaneous coronary procedures in the long term [7]. However, a prerequisite for successful percutaneous interventions in elderly patients is an experienced team of interventionists and a hospital where the treatment of elderly patients with coronary heart disease is routine [8].

■ Invasive investigation and interventional treatment of coronary heart disease in elderly patients in Switzerland

In Switzerland, as in other European countries, there are hardly any studies of invasive investigation and interventional treatment of elderly patients with coronary heart disease, which present hard evidence to confirm the superiority of this procedure compared to a more conservative strategy with drug treatment. However, such studies are needed urgently, since the numbers of procedures performed on elderly patients are increasing rapidly, although it is unclear whether a better relationship of effort and benefit with regard to prognosis, quality of life and costs can be achieved. We therefore carried out the first randomised Swiss multicentre study of the treatment of coronary heart disease in patients over 75 years, with a primary end point of quality of life, comparing the more aggressive invasive interventional strategy with the conservative medical strategy. A pilot project carried out in 4 hospitals with very active cardiac catheterisation laboratories (Universitätsklinik Basel, Herzzentrum Bad Krozingen, Hôpital Colmar and Mulhouse) in 183 patients aged over 75 years who had coronary angiography because of coronary heart disease showed that the proportion of women was greater in this group at 45% than in younger groups and that there is a relatively frequent (37%) previous history of a myocardial infarction. 61% had hypertension or dyslipidaemia, 21% were smokers, and 17% had diabetes mellitus. 74% of the patients had angina pectoris of NYHA $\geq$ III and 40% suffered from dyspnoea $>$ NYHA grade II. The angiographic findings showed single vessel disease in 26%, double vessel disease in 22% and triple vessel disease in 38%. 13% did not have a stenosis of the coronary arteries greater than 50%. A stenosis responsible for the current symptoms was located in the anterior interventricular branch in 27%, in the RCA in 24%, in the circumflex artery in 14% and in the left main stem in 3%. In 31%, a "culprit lesion" could not be defined and in 1% a high-grade stenosis in a vein bypass was the cause of the angina. In this pilot project, the therapeutic decisions in each hospital were made in accordance with local practice.

A correspondingly higher percentage of revascularisation procedures was preformed depending on the aggressiveness of the interventional team and cardiac surgery (Universitätsklinik Basel 68%, Hôpitaux Colmar/Mulhouse 62%, Bad Krozingen 37%). Within the pilot project, 46% of the patients who had invasive investigation were treated medically, 39% had a percutaneous coronary intervention and 13% underwent aortocoronary bypass surgery. In the course of the following 6 months, an ischaemic event occurred significantly more often in the medically treated group (61% conservative versus 10% PCI versus 16% CABG), while further revascularisation procedures were more frequent in the PCI group (35% PCI versus 0% medical treatment and CABG). The improvement in quality of life was markedly better with revascularisation than with medical treatment alone, while worsening of the quality of life was reported more often with medical treatment. The results of this pilot study showed that revascularisation can be performed in the majority of patients over 75 years with high-grade angina, which contributes on the one hand to the prevention of ischaemic events and also to an improvement in the quality of life in the next 6 months. These results reinforced endeavours to carry out the planned randomised Swiss multicentre study TIME (Trial of Invasive versus Medical Therapy in the Elderly).

▨ Trial of invasive versus medical therapy in the elderly (TIME, Swiss multicentre study)

Patients aged ≥75 years with angina pectoris of CCS class II–IV despite medical anti-ischaemic treatment with at least 2 drugs were included in the TIME study. Exclusion criteria are comorbidity with severely limited prognosis, unstable angina refractory to treatment, an acute myocardial infarction within the previous 10 days, severe aortic stenosis and absence of patient consent. The end points of this study, which is to include 300 patients, are quality of life, death, ischaemic events, hospitalisations and costs. The patients are randomised to a conservative medical arm and an arm with coronary angiography, interventional or surgical revascularisation. The follow-up is 6 months. The inclusion phase will be concluded in November 2000, and the results are expected in summer 2001 (ESC Meeting 2001).

▨ Acute coronary syndrome in elderly patients in Switzerland

As part of the MACS (Management in Acute Coronary Syndrome) project, a prospective register was drawn up in 25 hospitals in Switzerland of the current treatment of acute coronary syndrome. In the period from June 1998 to April 1999, 121 patients with unstable angina and 50 patients with non-Q wave myocardial infarction were included.

The median age was 65 (range 37–87) years, and 23% were women. Of the women, 37% were over 75 years, 24% were between 65 and 74 years and 39% were under 64 years old. The corresponding age cohorts in the men were 17%, 31% and 52%. When the frequency with which an invasive procedure was selected in patients under and over 64 years with acute coronary syndrome was compared, it was apparent that the invasive procedure was chosen in 25% of the older patient group and in 44% of the younger patient group. However, if an invasive investigation was chosen, an interventional or surgical revascularisation was performed more frequently in the elderly patient group (92% versus 66%) [9]. There is therefore still an inhibitory threshold in elderly patients for diagnosing acute coronary heart disease by invasive means. Those patients in whom coronary angiography was finally performed nearly all underwent revascularisation.

■ Summary

The risk of complications with percutaneous coronary interventions increases with age. In the past, elderly patients with coronary artery disease have therefore been excluded from randomized trials comparing conservative and interventional treatment strategies. Thus, hard evidence promoting an interventional strategy in this age group is lacking. Smaller studies have shown a similar gain in quality of life and functional status after percutaneous coronary interventions in elderly versus younger patients with coronary artery disease. In Switzerland, an increasing number of elderly patients with coronary artery disease is undergoing percutaneous coronary interventions. Nevertheless, invasive investigations of elderly patients with acute coronary syndromes still appears to be underused although a larger proportion of such patients will undergo revascularisation in comparison to younger patients. The inclusion phase of a larger randomized multicentre trial in Switzerland (TIME) in elderly patients with stable coronary artery disease was recently completed. Quality of life will be compared between the invasive and the conventional group during a follow-up of 6 months. The results are to be presented at the ESC meeting 2001.

■ References

1. Lindsay J Jr, Reddy VM, Pinnow EE, Little T, Pichard AD (1994) Morbidity and mortality rates in elderly patients undergoing percutaneous coronary transluminal angioplasty. Am Heart J 128:697–702
2. Statistisches Jahrbuch Schweiz. Bundesamt für Statistik, Bern (1990)
3. Elveback LR, Connolly DC, Melton LJ (1986) Coronary heart disease in residents of Rochester, Minnesota. IVV. Incidence, 1950 through 1982. Mayo Clin Proc 61:896–900
4. Ladwig KH, Scheuermann W (1994) Gender differences in the decline of mortality rates of acute myocardial infarction in West Germany. Eur Heart J 18:582–587
5. Gersh BJ, Kronmal RA, Frey RL, Schaff HV, Ryan TJ, Gosselin AJ, Kaiser GC, Killip T (1983) Coronary arteriography and coronary artery bypass surgery: morbidity and mortality in patients ages 65 years or older. A report from the Coronary Artery Surgery Study. Circulation 67:483–491

6. Seto TB, Taira DA, Berenzin R, Chauhan MS, Cutlip DE, Ho KKL, Kuntz RE, Cohen DJ (2000) Percutaneous coronary revascularization in elderly patients: Impact on functional status and quality of life. Ann Intern Med 132:955–958
7. Krumholz HM, Forman DE, Kuntz RE, Baim DS, Wei JY (1993) Coronary revascularization after myocardial infarction in the very elderly: outcomes and long-term follow-up. Ann Intern Med 119:1084–1090
8. Jollis JG, Peterson ED, Nelson CL, Stafford JA, DeLong ER, Lawrence HM, Mark DB (1997) Relationship between physician and hospital coronary angioplasty volume and outcome in elderly patients. Circulation 95:2485–2491
9. Remondino A, Amann FW, Bertel O, Erne P, Meier B, Angehrn W, Buser P (2000) Ist die invasive Abklärung von "älteren" Patienten mit akutem Koronarsyndrom sinnvoll? Kardiovask Med 3:S32

▪ Koronarinterventionen beim alten Menschen – Schweizer Sicht

P. BUSER

Das Komplikationsrisiko bei invasiven, interventionellen und chirurgischen Eingriffen ist bei über 75-jährigen Patienten größer als bei jüngeren Patienten. Der Erfolg einer Revaskularisation insbesondere in Bezug auf die Lebensqualität ist bei beiden Patientenpopulationen vergleichbar. Randomisierte Studien zum Vergleich eines invasiven versus eines konservativ medikamentösen Vorgehens bei älteren Patienten mit stabiler Angina pectoris liegen noch nicht vor. Im Sommer 2001 sind aus der TIME-Studie neue Erkenntnisse zu erwarten. Bei den akuten Koronarsyndromen besteht in der Schweiz immer noch ein großer Vorbehalt, ältere Patienten früh invasiv abzuklären, obwohl – wenn abgeklärt – viel häufiger als bei jüngeren Patienten eine Revaskularisation durchgeführt wird.

CHAPTER 4 Cardiac surgery in the elderly

R. S. HARTZ

Cardiothoracic surgery in very elderly patients is a major medical problem in the United States. In a recent state of the union address, President Clinton addressed the aging population as America's biggest priority, and a review of America's changing demographics reinforces his observation. The first "baby boomer" (a group that includes President Clinton) will reach age 65 in the year 2011. There will be an increasingly large group of patients who will need all forms of medical and surgical therapies in the very near future. One in five Americans will reach Medicare age 30 years from now, half of our current population will reach the octogenarian age level, and 19 million Americans will be greater than age 85 by the year 2050. Even more astounding is the fact that we currently have 61000 centenarians but that number will increase to a million in 30 years (Table 1) [1]. It is clear that the practice of medicine must change dramatically to accommodate these extremely elderly patients. For that reason the Society of Thoracic Surgeons is one of many organizations that have become involved in a cooperative effort with the American Geriatrics Society.

The issue of "how old is old?" is a difficult one. According to Satchell Paige, "how old would you be if you didn't know how old you were?"

Table 1. The aging population

Medicare patients
– First baby boomers in 2011
– 1/5 in 2030 bs. 1/11 in 1968
Octogenarians
– Half of population will reach
– 19 million $\geq$ 85 in 2050
Centenarians
– 61000 in 1998
– 1 million in 2030

Table 2. "Old" – millenium definition

■ 65 = middle-aged
■ 70 = elderly
■ 75 = old
■ 85 = "oldest-old"

In the words of this writer, "It is never too late to have a happy child-hood." More scientifically, a survey of the available literature was under-taken in order to determine the accurate definition of "old" today. Clearly 65 is not "old" but currently qualifies as "declining middle-age". If one reviews a surgical series that describes 65-year-olds in my speci-alty, the conclusions may be completely irrelevant as such patients are now young in many of our practices. There appears to be no debate that age 70 is classified as "elderly" in the medical and surgical litera-ture, that at age 75 a patient can probably be accurately classified as "old" and at age 85 the term "oldest-old" is being used increasingly in geriatric, surgical, and medical literature (Table 2). The only term that is not fully addressed here and is more illusive is the term "afraid el-derly." Obviously some patients as young as age 50 can be placed in this latter classification, especially when they are long-term diabetics, but the term is being used with increasing frequency as each decade of life passes, even in patients without co-morbid conditions.

American citizens have definite preferences concerning their categor-ization. In a recent article in Gerontologist, Chafetz et al. surveyed nu-merous geriatric patients in order to determine what they preferred to be called. These people hate the terms "old man/old woman or older person," detest "old timer and geezer" and even dislike "aging" and "geriatric." They prefer the nouns "senior citizen, retiree, senior, older adult," and the adjective "mature" [5]. Moreover, as life expectancy in-creases in this country, the definition is a moving target.

The background behind this presentation came when the John Hart-ford Society, a $ 450 million company specifically interested in geriatric research, allocated $ 17 million for various grants in care of the elderly, especially that provided by nurses and physicians. An increasing num-ber of such grants are now available for geriatric studies in all fields of medicine. The surgical specialties first became involved in the efforts of the Hartford Society in 1994 when a series of conferences was held and personnel was assembled to administer the grant funds. Five specialties were targeted in Phase I, one being general surgery and, largely due to the pioneering efforts of Dr. Walter Pories, an extensive core curriculum for education of surgical residents in geriatric principles was rapidly developed. Also, good literature, such as a frequently quoted multi-centre randomized trial of laparoscopic cholecystectomy in octogenarians [15] began to be published. Phase II of the Hartford project began in 1997 when project partners were named and five new specialties, including cardiothoracic surgery, were targeted. Seed grants were also established for institutions wishing to add geriatric topics to the curricula. The actual involvement of thoracic surgery in this effort began in May of 1998 when this author was appointed by the Society of Thoracic Surgeons (STS) to attend a conference in upstate New York. Clearly, we were "the new kids on the block." Although we had done very little background work, we were able to organize a symposium on geriatric care in cardiothoracic patients by the January 1999 meeting of the STS. This presentation is a summary of the cardiac portion of that conference.

There is a critical shortage of geriatric specialists in America and the specialty itself has not yet been elevated to the prestige and sophistication of pediatrics or internal medicine. There were only 8800 certified geriatricians (i.e., board certified or certificates of competence in geriatrics) in the year of 1998. It has been estimated that to continue to care for our aging population we will need 36000 geriatricians by the year of 2030, clearly an unreachable goal. There simply are not enough training programs. We must, therefore, increase geriatric knowledge in all other specialties. The few board-certified geriatricians should be doing geriatric research, dealing with critically ill patients such as those iatrogenically over medicated ("polypharmacy patients"), studying methods to improve inpatient and outpatient geriatric care on other services (including "house calls"), and educating physicians in other specialties about geriatric problems. Only 3% of American medical school graduates have any geriatric training and there are about 500 jobs available per geriatric trainee. We clearly do not have too many doctors in America but simply an imbalance between primary care and specialty physicians.

A fundamental issue that must be addressed is the question "does greater longevity mandate greater disability?" If our population is to age more and better, what will be the eventual outcome? There is a good range of data to help us answer this question. For example, a recent report from the New England Journal of Medicine involved a survey of 1741 university graduates. The study was conducted at Stanford University and the patients were surveyed annually from 1962 to 1994. Those patients at "high health risk" at baseline and in the early 1980s (defined as smoking, inactivity, and high body mass index) had significantly greater disability. What was unique about the Stanford study was that patients with low health risk at baseline experienced five additional years without significant disability, and lived five years longer than those with high health risk scores [24]. Thus, our efforts to exercise, not smoke, and be thin may indeed lead to longer and better lives.

Another significant, and even more difficult question is "what do our elderly patients want?" Do they *want* intensive care? Do they *want* to have high risk surgical procedures? The hospitalized elderly longitudinal project (HELP Study) is a study that used an approach called "value assessment" to determine the desires of elderly patients concerning their health care. In the United States, health values are used not only to determine clinical policy but also to dictate health care policy at the national level (making studies such as this one timely and crucial). The value assessment evaluated in this study was that of "time trade-off," essentially a measure of quantity vs. quality of life. Participants were asked "how much time would you give up in your current state of health for a period of time in excellent health?" There were 1266 patients, all 80 or older. Of the group, 414 were able to complete the baseline survey, which included understanding all tests and questions and in addition having a surrogate (spouse, friend, significant other, or care giver) who could also complete the survey. For the 414 patients baseline interviews were completed by both patient and surrogate. Twelve months later 176 patients and surrogates repeated the survey. The results were somewhat surprising. A full 40% of patients were unwilling to trade *any* time in their current state of health for a period of time in good health. Of the remaining 60%, one-third were willing to give up one month of life for a period of time in excellent health and a very small percent preferred just two weeks of excellent health to their current state of health. Overall the group equated one year of their current health to 9.7 months of excellent health. The answers of the proxies or the surrogates were not useful nor was any form of statistical manipulation (including multivariate analysis). The investigators concluded that these patients had a "strong will-to-live" even at age 80 or greater [23].

Why is the geriatric effort so important in cardiac surgery? Table 3 answers this question. Ischemic heart disease is the number one cause of both mortality and morbidity in American octogenarians and significantly effects 20% of that population. Twenty percent need some form of therapy; medical, surgical, or interventional. Given the number of octogenarians in the US, the number of health care dollars needed to care for these patients is staggering, and the number of health care givers necessary is also daunting. It is important to examine whether medical or surgical therapy offers any particular advantages to the

Table 3. IHD in octogenarians

▪ Leading cause of mortality and morbidity

▪ Affects 20%

▪ Medical Rx (76%)
  - 30-day mortality (no catheterization) 16%
  - 30-day mortality (after catheterization) 25%
  - 1-year survival 82%
  - 1-year event-free 55%
  - 50% in angina class III–IV

elderly population. For octogenarians with significant IHD who are treated medically (75% of the group), the 30-day mortality rate of those who do not undergo cardiac catheterization is 16%, and of the patients who have coronary angiography another 25% die within 30 days. Overall survival at one year is 82% but the event-free survival rate (no infarction, angina, stroke, or hospitalization) is only 55% and half of the patients are in angina class III–IV at one year [14]. Quality of life concerns, therefore, mandate that physicians at least *consider* interventional therapy or surgery in these patients.

Data concerning a coronary angioplasty (PTCR or percutaneous transluminal coronary revascularization) in American octogenarians arc almost impossible to obtain. For example, the American College of Cardiology (ACC) angioplasty database is voluntary and used by very few institutions. In 1996 only 137,000 patients who had coronary angiography and 125000 who had angioplasty were entered (personal communication). Since in that same year 300000 underwent bypass surgery there is clearly a need to improve on voluntary reporting of catheterization and angioplasty. The mean ages of patients entered in the ACC registry were 62.9 and 62.6 respectively for cardiac catheterization and angioplasty. Furthermore, the cut-off age for most interventional trials is 65. These facts make direct comparisons of surgery and angioplasty very difficult. In contrast the STS coronary bypass database (also voluntary) currently contains almost a million patients. The mean age of patients increased from 64 in the first year of data entry (1990) to 64.8 in 1997 (in 1980 mean age was 58.5) (Table 4). A more detailed analysis of the 1996 data revealed that 25% of patients were women, and 8% were non-Caucasian. The mean age of male Caucasian patients was 63.9, male non-Caucasian 61.9, female Caucasian 64.4, and female non-Caucasian 67.4. Although the STS database has the same flaws inherent as any other voluntary database, and is composed largely of

Table 4. Age of CABG patients (STS National Cardiac Database)

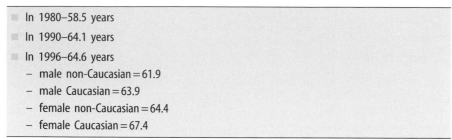

- ▦ In 1980–58.5 years
- ▦ In 1990–64.1 years
- ▦ In 1996–64.6 years
  - – male non-Caucasian = 61.9
  - – male Caucasian = 63.9
  - – female non-Caucasian = 64.4
  - – female Caucasian = 67.4

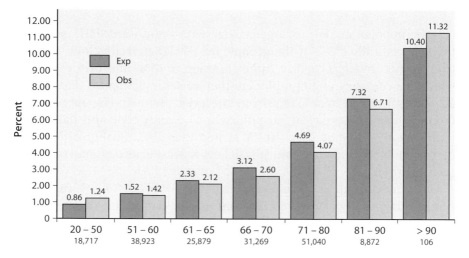

Fig. 1. Operative mortality by age group. US data 1997 CAB (N = 174 806)

male-Caucasian patients, the sheer number of patients studied (over half of CABG procedures in America entered in the last several years) make it a powerful tool for analyzing surgical outcomes in these various subpopulations.

The data shown in Fig. 1 [7] represent outcomes of patients having CABG in 1997. It is both impressive and intimidating since observed mortality rates are so low, especially in patients younger than age 80. This information is readily available to American hospitals and the media, and encourages surgical programs to turn down high-risk patients. Note particularly the observed mortality of 6.7% in octogenarians and 11.3% in nonogenarians, but cardiac surgery programs in America are expected to have an approximately 3% overall mortality rate for CABG. Individual CABG series almost invariably provide different data than does the STS database. For a group of 306 septuagenarians, Parry et al.

Table 5. Medicare database (N = 24 461)

	Age 65–70	Age ≥ 80
30-day mortality	4.3%	10.5%
1-year mortality	7.9%	19.3%
3-year mortality	13.1%	28.5%

quoted a mortality rate similar to STS databases (6.9%) but the difference between elective and emergency mortality was significantly different (1.9% vs. 16.7%) [18]. Emergency operation in elderly patients often carries a prohibitive risk not only in bypass surgery, but in noncardiac thoracic and general surgery. For example, emergency operation in 80-year-old patients was an independent risk factor for mortality after laparoscopic cholecystectomy [15]. Katz et al. demonstrated that age 70 is the cut-off for significant increases in hospital and 30-day mortality, and in hospital length of stay [11].

One of the first studies that pointed out the impact of gender on operative mortality in septuagenarians was that of Gehlot et al. who observed that operative mortality in 170 patients was 2.9%. Elective, urgent, and emergency operation (the latter defined as CABG on same day as cardiac catheterization) led to 2.1%, 3.1%, and 11.1% mortality respectively. Female gender was also a predictor of mortality in this series [8]. In a larger study (almost 700 patients) Curtis showed that mortality was significantly greater in women over age 70 (p < 0.005) [6].

The Medicare database is not voluntary and includes the records of all hospitalized patients older than age 65. For almost 25 000 CABG patients significant differences were noted in the 65 to 70-year-old and the greater than 80-year-old cohorts. Thirty-day mortality was 4.3% for the former and 10.5% for the latter. The one- and three-year mortality rates for octogenarians were similar to those of the general population indicating that not only symptom relief but also survival benefit can be obtained by treating octogenarians with CABG (Table 5) [19]. Unfortunately, the published Medicare data do not allow a breakdown of patients in their seventies, to determine the exact age at which operative risk increased.

As the age of patients in CABG series increases, so does the percentage of women. Cane et al. reported that of 121 octogenarians whose operation included CABG, 45% were women. A retrospective analysis of their medical records revealed that operative mortality was 9.1%. Follow-up information was obtained by phone contact with the patient, a family member, or the managing physician. Actual survival was 32.8%, compared to 37.6% for an age, gender, and race-matched population. Thus, CABG provided better quality of life, and also prolonged survival in this group of patients [4]. It is extremely important to operate on this elderly group in an elective setting. Williams and co-authors, who encourage referral of very old patients to their surgical program, noted an 11% operative mortality in 300 consecutive octogenarians undergoing elective CABG, but 30% mortality in those who underwent an emergency CABG (i.e., performed on the same day as the cardiac catheterization) [25].

Quality of care measures have become increasingly important as the age of patients undergoing CABG increases. Of particular importance is the frequent quote that the STS data *prove* that use of the left internal mammary artery (LIMA) improves operative mortality and long-term survival. Although the data are compelling, no such cause-and-effect relationship has ever been statistically established. Frequently (in 40% of data forms) the IMA data are incomplete. LIMA use increased in STS patients from 48.5% in 1990 to 79.8% in 1997, and overall mortality decreased. In septuagenarians, Azariades et al. used the LIMA in 33% of patients in whom operative mortality was 2.8% in contrast to 7.6% in those who did not have an IMA graft. There may have been selection bias, but five-year survival was also better in those patients with an IMA graft (89% vs. 78%) [3]. Clearly, other issues besides IMA use must be taken into consideration before proving that the conduit itself improves results. He et al. noted a highly significant difference in mortality in their patients younger than 70 (1.97%) and older than 70 (7.62%), all of whom had an IMA used. In univariate and logistic regression analysis, variables that predicted operative mortality included emergency operation, bilateral IMA use, and right internal mammary use (6.5% mortality with LIMA vs. 21.6% with RIMA). The authors concluded that use of the RIMA as a bypass conduit in the elderly should not yet be universally accepted [9]. In another fairly large series of octogenarians, Morris did not note a difference in mortality in octogenarians with and without an IMA (7.9% vs. 7%) but survival was better at two-, three-, and five-year follow up with the IMA use. He concluded that the LIMA as the bypass graft of choice "should not be denied to this high-risk group" [17].

I have previously referred to geriatrics as "the age of women" and there is no question that the bulk of American health care dollars used to treat ischemic heart disease will eventually be shifted to the female population. Women currently outlive men by 7.5 years. In addition, in the "oldest-old" group the female:male ratio is 2.2:1.0 [20]. In the STS database, the percentage of women increased only from 27.3% to 30%

Table 6. PTCR in 80-year-olds – meta-analysis

■ Mean-age = 83
■ ♂: ♀ equal
■ 83% clinical success
■ 7% hospital mortality (1–19)
■ 20% repeat revascularization

between 1990 and 1997 but this figure is likely to change significantly as the female population continues to live longer. Currently, the life expectancy of an octogenarian woman is 9.1 years and for men 7.0 years. Obviously, patients who need bypass surgery in this age group will be much sicker with multiple co-morbid conditions and higher acuity scores. The issue of interventional therapy (PTCR) vs. CABG will become increasingly relevant over the next decade or two, and many of these patients will automatically be referred to tertiary programs that encourage referral of high-risk patients.

In addition to the Medicare data on 20 000 angioplasty patients (7% mortality) a meta-analysis of eight series performed by Little and Lindsay (mean age of patients was 83 years) revealed that half of the patients were women, overall success rate was 83%, and hospital mortality was 7%. Twenty percent of patients required repeat revascularization within a year (Table 6) [14]. There have also been two single-center studies of angioplasty in octogenarians. Mick et al. reported 2% mortality in 53 interventional patients vs. 6% in 153 CABG patients in 1991 [16] and in 1994, in a larger group of patients (105 angioplasties, 205 CABG) Kaul et al. noted a *lower* mortality rate for CABG than for an angioplasty (5.8% vs. 8.6%). In his series, 71% of the PTCR patients and 46% of CABG patients were women. Both five-year and event-free survival were significantly greater in the surgical group. This study is frequently quoted because the surgical group was actually sicker than the angioplasty group but had better outcomes (Table 7) [12].

There is only a small amount of data available concerning quality of life after bypass surgery in elderly patients, but a few studies indicate that the procedure results in better functional class in septuagenarians [10], that an increasing number of octogenarians are happy with their decision to have undergone CABG [13], and that patients who accepted CABG had better three-year survival, better quality of life, and lower cost per "quality life-year" than those who refused CABG [21].

A brief discussion of less invasive surgical techniques is appropriate since procedures such as off pump CABG (OPCAB) and minimally in-

Table 7. PTCR vs. CABG in octogenarians

	PTCR	CABG
N	105	205
% women	71	46
% mortality	8.6	5.8
LOS	7	14*
% 5-year survival	55	66*
3 years event-free	61	81*

* p < 0.01

vasive CABG (MIDCAB) may be ideal for the "oldest-old" patients, especially those with significant atherosclerosis of the ascending aorta or with renal failure. Although MIDCAB is falling out of favor in America, Zenati et al. showed in 1997 that, in a group of 17 patients, all refused surgery elsewhere and referred to the University of Pittsburgh, there was no operative mortality, there were no strokes, and length of stay was 3.9 days. Of the 17 patients, 11 had MIDCAB alone and six had a hybrid procedure involving angioplasty [26]. More and more technical expertise, and increased collaboration between specialties, will undoubtedly result in improved outcomes and quality of life in our oldest citizens with ischemic heart disease.

To briefly address other types of cardiac surgery, aortic and mitral valve replacement are frequently recommended in elderly patients. Just as for CABG, the mean age for aortic valve replacement (AVR) patients has changed minimally in the STS database, from 64.3 years in 1990 to 65.4 in 1997. In contrast, results of surgery are distinctly different. In young patients (up to age 60) the mortality for AVR is slightly higher than for CABG (2.4% age 20–50, 3.1% age 50–60). However, in isolated AVR for aortic stenosis, the mortality rates are lower than for CABG (5.7% and 6.3% in octogenarians and nonogenarians respectively) [Fig. 2]. These numbers are even more impressive because re-do procedures are included in the analysis. The addition of CABG to an AVR procedure changes outcome significantly. In a large series of septuagenarians (n = 717, mean age 77 years), Aranki et al. achieved an overall mortality of 6.6% overall, but 4.2% for isolated AVR and 8.8% for AVR with CABG (p < 0.01). For women the differences were even greater, 2.9% mortality for AVR alone, but 10.3% for AVR with CABG. In men, the addition of CABG to an AVR procedure did not significantly affect operative outcomes. Thus gender, but not age, predicted mortality with combined AVR/CABG [2].

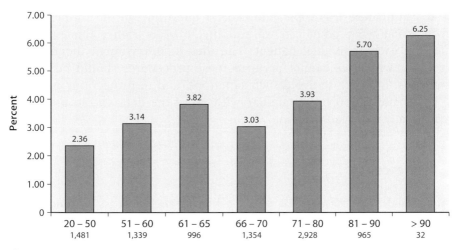

Fig. 2. Operative mortality by age group. US data 1997 aortic valve replacement (N = 9095)

Table 8. Heart surgery in octogenarians

▪ 528 consecutive patients
▪ 44% women
▪ Mortality rates (mean = 10.6%)
– CABG (303) = 8.3%
– AVR ± CABG (132) = 4.5%
– MVR ± CABG (42) = 29%
– M rep. ± CABG (31) = 23%
– DVR ± CABG (20) = 30%

The data for mitral valve replacement (MVR) are much different than for AVR. For isolated MVR, operative mortality in the STS database is higher than for CABG in both septuagenarians and octogenarians (9.5% and 14% respectively), and there are no patients older than age 90 in database. It is important to review individual series because there are so few very elderly patients undergoing MVR in the United States. Tsai et al. reported on heart surgery in 528 consecutive octogenarians in 1994. The overall mortality rate was 10.6%; for CABG 8.3%, for AVR with or without CABG 4.5%, for MVR with or without CABG 29%, and for double valve replacement with or without CABG 30% [22] (Table 8). Because of the extremely high operative mortality in these patients, it is even more important to carefully weigh the risk: benefit ratios, and to operate in an elective situation as often as possible.

To summarize this topic, the crucial question for the thoracic surgeon is "at what point can we add life to years rather than years to life?" in each individual patient. The idea of government dictating an age after which we cannot perform these procedures should be alarming to us. In order to avoid such sanctions, and to protect our patients, it is our obligation to be familiar with all of the data and to discuss it realistically with each patient.

■ References

1. Alexander KP, Peterson ED (1997) Coronary artery bypass grafting in the elderly. American Heart Journal 134:856–864
2. Aranki SF et al. (1993) Aortic valve replacement in the elderly. Effect of gender and coronary artery disease on operative mortality. Circulation 88:17–23
3. Azariades M et al. (1990) Five-year results of coronary bypass grafting for patients older than 70 years: role of internal mammary artery. Annals of Thoracic Surgery 50:940–945
4. Cane ME et al. (1995) CABG in octogenarians: early and late events and actuarial survival in comparison with a matched population. Annals of Thoracic Surgery 60:1033–1037
5. Chafetz PK et al. (1998) Older adults and the news media: utilization, opinions, and preferred reference terms. Gerontologist 38:481–489
6. Curtis JJ et al. (1995) Coronary revascularization in the elderly; determinants of operative mortality. Annals of Thoracic Surgery 58:1069–1072
7. Data Analyses of The Society of Thoracic Surgeons National Adult Cardiac Surgery Database (1998) Operative mortality by age group: 107, 113
8. Gehlot AS et al. (1994) Current status of coronary artery bypass grafting in patients 70 years of age and older. Australian & New Zealand Journal of Surgery 65:177–181
9. He GW et al. (1994) Determinants of operative mortality in elderly patients undergoing coronary artery bypass grafting. Emphasis on the influence of internal mammary artery grafting on mortality and morbidity. Journal of Thoracic & Cardiovascular Surgery 108:73–81
10. Jaeger AA et al. (1994) Functional capacity after cardiac surgery in elderly patients. Journal of the American College of Cardiology 24:104–108
11. Katz NM et al. (1995) Cardiac operations in patients aged 70 years and over: mortality, length of stay, and hospital charge. Annals of Thoracic Surgery 60:96–100
12. Kaul T et al. (1994) Angioplasty versus coronary artery bypass in octogenarians. Annals of Thoracic Surgery 58:1419–1426
13. Kumar P et al. (1995) Quality of life in octogenarians after open heart surgery. Chest 108:919–926
14. Little T, Lindsay J (1994) Percutaneous transluminal coronary angioplasty and coronary artery bypass graft surgery in octogenarians: indications and outcome. Heart Disease and Stroke 3:261–265
15. Maxwell JG et al. (1998) Laparoscopic cholecystectomy in octogenarians. American Surgeon 64:826–831

16. Mick MJ et al. (1991) Early and late results of coronary angioplasty and by-pass in octogenarians. American Journal of Cardiology 68:1316–1320
17. Morris RJ et al. (1996) Internal thoracic artery for coronary artery grafting in octogenarians. Annals of Thoracic Surgery 62:16–22
18. Parry AJ et al. (1994) An audit of cardiac surgery in patients aged over 70 years. Quarterly Journal of Medicine 87:89–96
19. Peterson ED et al. (1995) Outcomes of coronary artery bypass graft surgery in 24,461 patients 80 years or older. Circulation 92:85–91
20. Rochon P, Gurwitz J (1998) Geriatrics: the age of women. Lancet 348 (Suppl II) 8:9043
21. Sollano JA et al. (1998) Cost-effectiveness of coronary artery bypass surgery in octogenarians. Annals of Surgery 228:297–306
22. Tsai TP et al. (1994) Ten-year experience of cardiac surgery in patients aged 80 years and over. Annals of Thoracic Surgery 58:445–450
23. Tsevat J et al. (1998) Health values of hospitalized patients 80 years or older. JAMA 279:371–375
24. Vita AJ et al. (1998) Aging, health risks, and cumulative disability. New England Journal of Medicine 338:1035–1041
25. Williams DB et al. (1995) Determinants of operative mortality in octogenarians undergoing coronary bypass. Annals of Thoracic Surgery 60:1038–1043
26. Zenati M et al. (1998) Preoperative risk models for minimally invasive coronary bypass: a preliminary study. Journal of Thoracic & Cardiovascular Surgery 116:584–589

■ Herzchirurgie im Alter

R. HARTZ

Herzchirurgische Eingriffe in der Gruppe der „sehr alten" Patienten stellen in den Vereinigten Staaten (USA) ein wachsendes medizinisches Problem dar. Die Zahl der Patienten, die in naher Zukunft alle verfügbaren medizinischen und chirurgischen Therapiekonzepte in Anspruch nehmen muss, steigt ständig. Die Hälfte aller gegenwärtig lebenden Amerikaner wird das achtzigste Lebensjahr erreichen und mehr als 19 Mio. Amerikaner werden im Jahre 2050 älter als 85 Jahre sein. Noch verblüffender ist jedoch die Tatsache, dass sich die Zahl der gegenwärtig 61 000 lebenden Siebzigjährigen in dreißig Jahren auf über eine Million erhöhen wird. Die gängige medizinische Praxis muss sich dramatisch wandeln, um den Erfordernissen dieser extrem alten Patienten gerecht zu werden. Für die Herzchirurgie ergeben sich dabei besondere Anforderungen. Die ischämische Herzkrankheit stellt die Hauptursache für Mortalität und Morbidität unter den Achtzigjährigen dar und beeinträchtigt 20% dieser Population. 20% von diesen Patienten benötigen eine Therapieform: medizinisch, interventionell, chirurgisch. In Anbetracht der Anzahl Achtzigjähriger US-Bürger schwanken die für das Gesundheitssystem bereitgestellten Mittel und die Anzahl der benötigten Dienstleister wird nur zögerlich benannt. Entscheidend ist es, zu untersuchen, ob die medizinische oder chirurgische Therapie dieser Patientenpopulationen Vorteile im Detail bietet. Achtzigjährige mit signifikanter ischämischer Herzkrankheit und unter medikamentöser Therapie (75% dieser Gruppe) weisen eine 30-Tage-Mortalität von 16% ohne kardangiographische Diagnostik auf. Von den mittels Herzkatheter untersuchten Patienten versterben dennoch 25% innerhalb der ersten 30 Tage. Das Gesamt-1-Jahres-Überleben beträgt 82%, wobei jedoch die ereignisfreie Überlebensrate (kein Infarkt, keine Angina, kein Apoplex, keine Hospitalisation) nur 55% ausmacht und die Hälfte der Patienten Angina-pectoris-Beschwerden der Klasse AP III–IV aufweist. Zur Gewährleistung einer vertretbaren Lebensqualität dieser Patienten sollten interventionelle oder chirurgische Therapieformen in Betracht gezogen werden. Dem gegenüber stehen jedoch die alarmierenden Bemühungen der Regierung, eine feste Altersobergrenze für diese Therapieoptionen zu etablieren. Um solche Sanktionen zum Schutz unserer Patienten zu verhindern, ist es die Pflicht von uns Ärzten, mit den Daten vertraut zu sein und diese Ergebnisse offen mit dem einzelnen Patienten zu diskutieren.

CHAPTER **5** ## On the economics of medical innovation

P. ZWEIFEL

■ Introduction and overview

This contribution starts with a puzzle. Why is it that health insurers
and policy makers are afraid of medical innovation whereas technological innovation is considered the source of cost savings in the remainder
of the economy? To see that there is a puzzle here, it is sufficient to
take the example of computers. One generation ago, mainframe computers used to occupy an entire room that needed to be airconditioned.
Today, a laptop has more computing power than most of those computers while costing maybe 1% of their price. By way of contrast, health
insurers and policy makers sigh everytime when the media announce a
new medical technology.

In an attempt to explain this puzzle, the important distinction between product innovation and process innovation is introduced in the
next section. In the case of a process innovation, the same merchandise
or service is produced at a lower cost; in the case of a product innovation, the merchandise or service in question is provided with new quality attributes, possibly at an increased cost. It will then be shown that
while a good deal of process innovation occurs in the remainder of the
economy, the existence of health insurance serves to bias the mix between the two in favor of product innovation. Thus, the bias in favor of
cost-increasing product innovation in health care may explain why
technological innovation in medicine is viewed as a mixed blessing by
many. A separate section will be devoted to the specific issue of medical
innovation benefitting elderly patients. The amazing finding will be
that the most recent and costly medical technology is often applied to
patients with very short remaining life expectancy. This finding poses
another puzzle. Why should people want to invest heavily in health care
if the payback period to their investment is so short as it is? While several answers to this question exist, there are policy options to deal with
this apparent anomaly. The final section contains a survey and evalua-
tion of these options. While age-dependent rationing of medical ser-

vices is advocated in many quarters, economic theory suggests more efficient alternatives such as the development of insurance contracts that induce a more judicious use of medical innovation towards the end of human life.

■ The economic distinction between process and product innovation

In economic theory, it has become customary to distinguish between two types of innovation, process and product innovation (see Table 1). In the case of a process innovation, the merchandise or service in question is produced at a lower cost, which typically means that the production process occurs at a faster pace. For this reason, process innovation often meets with a good deal of resistance on the part of the work force. It may suffice for the reader to imagine the medical director of a hospital department ordering the use of a new therapy that does not improve the prospect of recovery but requires nursing staff to work faster. Such an innovation would certainly be greeted with much scepticism by staff. The same is true of firms in the remainder of the economy; it is the pressure of worldwide price competition that forces firms to adopt unpopular process innovations.

By way of contrast, the idea behind a product innovation is to add new quality attributes to a merchandise or service [1]. Since consumers are willing to pay for these attributes, the new product will fetch a higher price. However, this means that the cost of production may go up without the firm losing its competitiveness. A higher cost base provides employees with a margin of maneuver, which may be used for perks that make work life more pleasant such as the outsourcing of onerous tasks or hiring additional help, new machinery, or reduced work hours.

Table 1. Aspects of process and product innovation

Aspect	Process innovation	Product innovation
Basic idea	"The same but less costly, faster"	"New attributes, may also cost more"
Consumers' willingness to pay	Unchanged	Increased and enhanced by a limited monopoly (patents)
Response within the firm	Considerable resistance	Support
Market result	The mix of the two types of innovation depends on cost-benefit considerations on the part of consumers	

Admittedly, the two types of innovation occur often in a way that makes it difficult to distinguish them in actual medical practice [5]. Still, it has proven fruitful to distinguish the two types at the conceptual level because their consequences are different. Indeed, if a country is successful in launching product innovations, it can permit itself an increase in the cost of labor which is nothing but higher wages for its work force. However, since consumers' willingness to pay for improved quality attributes is always limited, firms also need to continually introduce process innovations as well.

▦ **Conclusion 1.** Firms compete with improved quality and lower price. This causes a certain mix of process and product innovation in a market economy subject to international competition.

▦ The impact of health insurance on the innovation mix

Health insurance has the effect of changing the mix between process and product innovation in the health care sector [7]. Quite likely, willingness-to-pay of consumers (who are patients or prospective patients in the present context) is higher to begin with. After all, product innovation in medicine means improved chances of recovery and even survival, features that are highly valued by most individuals. Nevertheless, health insurance serves to magnify this tendency in favor of product innovation in medicine (see Table 2).

Table 2. The specific influence of health insurance on the innovation mix

Influence	Process innovation	Product innovation
▦ **On patients**	Little interest, since minimal share in savings achieved	Very much interested; reduction of effective total cost possible [a]
▦ **On physicians, hospitals**	Little interest, since minimal share in savings achieved	Very much interested since new products are crucial for competition for patients
▦ **On suppliers of innovation (pharmaceuticals, diagnostics)**	Only interested if potential for cost reduction large	Given that the innovation is insured; market success almost guaranteed
Result	Health insurance biases the mix between the two types of innovation in favor of product innovation	

[a] For an explanation, see Table 3 below.

For simplicity, the argument will be based on the case of a fully insured patient, as is true of the public ward of a hospital in Switzerland. To the extent that there is copayment (10% on ambulatory care expenditure in Switzerland), the conclusions reached would have to be modified slightly.

Put very simply, a fully insured patient is not interested in process innovation in medicine at all. At the time when he or she decides to initiate a treatment episode, the health insurance premium is already paid, constituting a fixed cost that has no relevance for decision making any more. Indeed, it does not matter to the insured whether a medical therapy costs $ 1000 or $ 10000, the effective out-of-pocket-cost being zero at any rate.

For physicians and hospitals, it thus makes little sense to try to attract patients by offering a low price. Accordingly, they also have little incentive to adopt cost-reducing process innovations. Of course, this would change as soon as insurers have the right to engage in selective contracting, permitting them to seek out those providers that offer a favorable quality-price ratio.

This lack of interest in process innovations finally spills over to suppliers of medical innovation such as pharmaceutical companies. They are hesitant to invest in new products that promise to reduce the cost of service in hospitals and medical practices.

Things are entirely different in the case of product innovation. Given that they are fully insured, patients have every incentive to opt for the highest quality available since even the newest therapy has an out-of-pocket price of zero to them. Physicians and hospitals in their turn know full well that they can attract insured patients by offering the newest medical technology. Finally, it is easy for the suppliers to sell a product innovation. Once their product has made it on the formulary (the list of benefits paid by health insurance), its success in the market is almost guaranteed.

In summary, the very existence of health insurance imparts a bias in favor of product innovation to the health care sector with cost-saving process innovations getting short thrift. This only changes if insurers have the right of selective contracting permitting them to retain only those physicians and hospitals that excel by their favorable quality-cost ratio. A favorable ratio factors into a favorable quality-premium ratio with which a health insurer can compete in the market for members.

■ **Conclusion 2.** The existence of health insurance imparts a bias in favor of product rather than process innovation to medical care, which is most marked as long as there is no selective contracting.

Table 3. Medical innovation and effective cost to the insured

Existing product	$
Maximum willingness-to-pay of insured (assumed)	20
Maximum price of product on the market (assumed rate of coinsurance 10%)	200
Time cost to patient (assumed 1 h at $ 30)	30
Total effective cost to patient	**50**
Product innovation	
Maximum willingness-to-pay of insured (assumed)	25
Maximum price of product on the market (assumed rate of coinsurance of 10%)	250
Time cost to patient (assumed 0.5 h at $ 30)	15
Total effective cost to patient	**40**

Conclusion holds true also in the presence of a (small) copayment. This can be seen from the following example (Table 3). Initially, let a patient's maximum willingness-to-pay be $ 20, e.g., for a drug. With a rate of copayment of 10%, the price of the drug may be as high $ 200 because, in that case, the out-pocket-cost to the patient is precisely $ 20. Moreover, assume that the actual purchase and administration of the drug uses one hour's worth of patient time, which is valued at $ 30. Therefore, initially the effective cost of the therapy is $ 50 to the insured patient.

Now let there be a product innovation, with two effects. First, the maximum willingness-to-pay increases to $ 25 in view of improved quality attributes. Accordingly, the market price of the drug may rise to $ 250. For simplicity, assume that the manufacturer actually charges that maximum price. Second, another improved feature of the drug may well be its less frequent administration. Let the patient time needed drop from 1 h to 30 min. Accordingly, taking the new drug entails a time cost of $ 15 rather than $ 30 as before.

In this example, the total effective cost to the patient decreases from $ 50 to $ 40. Therefore, more patients are likely to demand the product innovation. At the same time, its money price (which must be reimbursed by health insurance) has increased, from $ 180 (90% of 200) to $ 270 (90% of 300). This simple example may explain why health insurers are so nervous about medical innovation.

▪ Medical innovation and the elderly

Insurers and policymakers are particularly sceptical when costly medical innovation is applied to elderly patients. Being beyond retirement age, these patients no longer contribute to the financing of health care, at least in systems financed by payroll taxes (such as in Germany). On the other hand, the cost of medical care seems to increase with age, implying that there will be a future cost explosion due to population aging.

However, research undertaken by health economists has consistently shown that the probability of initiating a treatment episode does not increase with age as soon as health status is controlled for statistically [3, 4], (Table 4). This is important because the initiation of a treatment episode is a decision taken by the patient largely uninfluenced by the physician. Thus, it truly reflects a moral hazard effect, which economic theory predicts as a consequence of insurance coverage. In fact, the ten-

Table 4. The (lacking) relationship between HCE and age

Observation	Theoretical interpretation	Implication for health policy
▪ The probability of initiating a treatment episode does *not* increase with age, given health status	▪ For given health status and insurance coverage, there is no ground to suspect increased moral hazard among the aged	▪ No justification for controlling moral hazard among the aged by, e.g., mandating increased cost sharing for aged insureds
▪ Medical expenditure per treatment episode increases with age	▪ The true source of moral hazard could be the physician, who adjusts practice style to age (possibly in collusion)	▪ Make physicians participate in the financial result of the insurer (HMOs, houses for physicians)
	▪ Aging of population results in a future cost explosion!	▪ Limit treatment alternatives available to aged patients
▪ Medical expenditure increases sharply with closeness to death	▪ Not a sensible investment of resources since payback period short	▪ Age-dependent rationing of medical care (especially costly product innovations)
▪ Medical expenditure increases sharply with closeness to death *regardless* of age	▪ Reflects tendency towards "heroic efforts" on the part of physician	▪ No justification for age-dependent rationing
	▪ Reflects fear of death on the part of patient as the cause of extreme moral hazard	▪ Self-rationing of insureds through their choice of plan as an alternative

dency of insureds (noted in section 3 above) to opt for the newest and most expensive medical technology is nothing but a (dynamic) moral hazard effect, caused by the insureds being fully protected against the financial consequence of such a choice. For health policy, the absence of a relationship between age and HCE undermines the idea of controlling moral hazard specifically among the aged. For example, one might have argued in favor of increased cost sharing by the aged in an attempt to control their moral hazard.

Given that a treatment episode is initiated, the question still remains whether HCE increases with age on average. Health economics research has shown that there is a clear age effect, which may already mirror the influence of the physician adjusting his or her practice style to age. This adjustment could occur in collusion with the patient, thus reflecting moral hazard once more. For this reason, the aging of the population seems to result in a future cost explosion.

One way to counteract this tendency is to make physicians participate in the financial result of the insurer. This is what Health Maintenance Organisations (HMOs) and more generally bonuses for physicians paid for non-incurred HCE do. Another policy response is to limit the treatment alternatives available to elderly patients, which already amounts to a form of rationing.

More recent research, starting with that done by Lubitz and Prihoda [2] using US Medicare data, has found that HCE increases sharply with closeness to death. From an economic point of view, this is puzzling because lavishing resources shortly before death does not seem a sensible investment since the payback period is so short. One may, of course, resort to fear of death to explain this phenomenon. The implication for health policy of such behavior is clear: it provides the justification for age-dependent rationing of medical care, especially of costly product innovations.

Some very recent research suggests that the relationship between HCE and closeness to death is independent of the age of the individual [6]. Indeed, drawn from a sample of Swiss deceased, the evidence points to a reduction of HCE with closeness to death among individuals aged 65. The theoretical interpretation of this finding is that "heroic efforts" on the part of the physician occur to save the life of a death-bound person. It also may reflect fear of death on the part of the patient, implying an extremely strong moral hazard effect.

From the policy point of view, there is no reason any more for a future cost explosion due to aging (at least at the level of the individual). Whereas at present, the two expensive last years of life occur at ages 75/76 on average, in the future they may occur at ages 85/86, implying no more than that the costly phase of human life is deferred by ten years. Such a deferral, however, provides no justification for age-dependent rationing. Age-dependent rationing would also appear to be unfair because at age 70 (say), one individual may have a remaining life expectancy of only one year whereas another still has one of ten years.

However, the issue remains that individuals who presumably know that their remaining life expectancy is short nonetheless spend such a great deal on medical care, which is paid by others. The solution might be to induce self-rationing on the part of the aged by making them choose an insurance plan that imposes restrictions on the use of medical care – in return for a reduced contribution, of course. These policy options are expounded in the next section.

■ Reform options

Clearly, medical innovation poses a problem both to insurers and policy makers. The preferred policy choice in dealing with this problem has been the planning of innovation by public authorities or by a cartel of health insurers. For example, the public authority may state its intention to only finance so many MRIs per 10000 population. Social health insurers, acting as a cartel, can impose similar restrictions (see Table 5). Such planning certainly has its advantages. In particular, it makes

Table 5. Reform options for the management of medical innovation

Alternative	Advantages	Disadvantages
Planning of innovation by public authorities or by cartel of health insurers	Future health care expenditure easier to control by health insurers	Deteriorating benefit-cost ratios in the long run; loss of competitiveness of health care system
Health insurance plans that include medical innovations only when having demonstrated efficiency (in return for reduced contributions)	Permits consumers to express their individual preferences; provides partial escape from the "cost escalator"	Frequent regret of earlier decision, in particular
Health insurance plans selecting innovations for which willingness-to-pay is high	Insurance benefits structured according to consumer preferences; insurer balances benefits and costs (i.e., additional premium) on behalf of consumers	Challenge to the holders of incumbent slots in the catalog of benefits

controlling future HCE much easier for health insurers (or public authorities).

However, it also has important disadvantages. Since public planning does not take into account consumer preferences, the health care sector delivers less value for money, being too expensive for what it provides. Thus, benefit-cost ratios in health care deteriorate on the long run, causing a loss of competitiveness of the country's health care system and of the economy as a whole.

However, planning of medical innovation could be done by the individual insurer itself, acting on behalf of its clientele. For example, insurers could launch plans that only include medical innovations of demonstrated efficiency, in return for a reduced contribution. If they are subject to competition for members, they must pattern their benefits according to member preferences. Thus, consumers can express their individual preferences by their choice of plan. For those who do not want to pay the higher premium for having the latest medical technology included in the benefit package, a plan with delayed access to such technology would provide a partial escape from the "cost escalator" driven by product innovation in health care.

Such self-selected restrictions certainly have their disadvantages, too. In particular, insureds will frequently regret their past decisions. It may well be that when approaching death, many would want to have access to the latest medical technology in spite of earlier commitments to the contrary. However, scope for regret is the necessary correlate of free choice. For example, individuals make long-term commitments in their choice of occupation, marriage partner, and family size. These decisions can be changed at considerable cost – if at all. Yet, the freedom of individual choice is preserved in these domains.

One might ask the question of how insurers are able to structure their benefit packages on behalf of their members. Here, recent developments in experimental economics offer some good news. Willingness-to-pay for medical innovation can, for example, be estimated using a so-called Conjoint Analysis. This is a tool that has been developed in marketing. Respondents are faced with a series of scenarios where treatment alternatives vary in terms of their quality attributes (such as pain, probability of success, and amenities, and out-of-pocket price to the patient). All respondents have to do is to accept or reject a particular combination of attributes. From the responses, trade-offs can be filtered out which indicate the willingness-to-pay for a particular attribute. The total willingness-to-pay for a treatment can then be estimated by combining the different attributes. In this way, insurers will in the future be able to structure their benefits according to the preferences of their members. Their objective will be to balance the benefits against the costs (i.e., additional premium) on behalf of consumers. Admittedly, this development is likely to be slow because the holders of slots in the existing state of benefit package (especially in social insurance) will be challenged. Thus, they have little interest in having members' willing-ness-to-pay revealed.

■ **Conclusion 3.** The response to costly medical innovation benefitting in particular elderly patients need not be rationing and public planning. There are more consumer-friendly alternatives such as health insurance plans offering increased cost sharing beyond a certain age to contain moral hazard of offering delayed access to newest medical technology, both in return for reduced contributions.

Weeding out benefit packages from products that do not provide value for money is in the best long-run interest of the health care sector be-cause it fosters its competitiveness. Indeed, the economy as a whole profits from such a process because it too gains in competitiveness.

■ Conclusion

This contribution started with a puzzle. Why is it that innovation is viewed as progress in the remainder of the economy while being so much feared in the health care sector? The answer to this question seems to lie in a distinction between process innovation (which is cost-reducing) and product innovation (which is quality improvement but may be cost-in-creasing). Next, it was shown that the very existence of health insurance biases the mix of the two types of innovation in favor of product innova-tion. This bias becomes the more problematic as evidence accumulates that the latest medical technology is applied to patients that are in their last quarter of human life. Accordingly, even countries with a market economy have resorted to a public regulation of innovation in the health care sector. However, there are market-oriented alternatives: specifically, competing health insurers could be encouraged to develop new types of policies that give insureds access to new medical technologies only with a delay. In the meantime, their benefit-cost ratio can be established. In this way, medical innovation is tied more closely to the preferences of consumers, which can be measured in the guise of willingness-to-pay, using modern tools of experimental economics.

The requirement that health insurers are competing merits emphasis at this point. If permitted to act as a cartel, health insurers will not differ much from politicians because they collectively do not have to re-spect the preferences of their clients. Thus, countries that have initiated market-oriented reforms of their health care sectors (such as the Netherlands, Germany, and Switzerland) must pay increased attention to their competition policies with regard to health insurance.

■ References

1. Lancaster K (1971) Consumer Demand: A New Approach: Columbia University Press, New York
2. Lubitz J, Prihoda R (1984) Use and costs of Medicare services in the last years of life. In: Health Care Financing Review 5 (1), Spring, 117–131
3. Newhouse JP, Phelps ChE (1976) New estimates of price and income elasticities of medical care services. In: Rosett RN (ed) The Role of Health Insurance in the Health Services Sector. National Bureau of Economic Research, New York, 261–312
4. Newhouse JP, the Insurance Experiment Group (1993) Free for All? Lessons from the RAND Health Insurance Experiment. Harvard University Press, Cambridge MA
5. Zweifel P, Breyer F (1997) Health Economics. Oxford University Press, New York, pp 20–43
6. Zweifel P, Felder S, Meier M (2000) Aging of population and health care expenditure: a red herring? In: Health Economics 8 (6):485–496
7. Zweifel P, Manning WG (2000) Moral hazard and consumer incentives in health care. In: Culyer AJ, Newhouse JP (eds) Handbook of Health Economics. Elsevier, Boston, Ch. 8

▪ Ökonomische Aspekte medizinischer Innovationen

P. Zweifel

Dieser Beitrag geht von einem Rätsel aus: Warum fürchten die Krankenversicherer und Politiker die medizinische Innovation, wo doch technologische Innovation als die Quelle von Kosteneinsparungen in der übrigen Wirtschaft gilt? Zur Erklärung wird die Unterscheidung zwischen Produkt- und Prozessinnovation eingeführt. Im Falle einer Prozessinnovation wird das gleiche Gut oder die gleiche Dienstleistung zu niedrigeren Kosten hergestellt. Im Falle einer Produktinnovation hingegen wird das Gut oder die Dienstleistung mit neuen Qualitätseigenschaften versehen, was die Zahlungsbereitschaft der Käufer erhöht, sodass die Produktionskosten zunehmen dürfen. Es stellt sich heraus, dass die Krankenversicherung im Gesundheitswesen die Mischung zwischen diesen beiden Innovationstypen systematisch zu Gunsten der Produktinnovation verändert. Diese Verschiebung erklärt, weshalb medizintechnologische Innovationen von vielen mit gemischten Gefühlen betrachtet werden. Der Beitrag geht auch auf das besondere Problem von medizinischen Innovationen zugunsten älterer Patienten ein. Tatsächlich wird ja die neueste und kostspieligste Technologie öfter an Patienten angewendet, die lediglich eine sehr kurze Lebenserwartung haben. Dies führt zu einem zweiten Rätsel: Warum investieren Individuen so viel in Gesundheitsleistungen, wenn die sog. Rückzahlungsdauer einer solchen Investition dermaßen kurz ist? Darauf gibt es noch keine eindeutige Antwort; dennoch bestehen Möglichkeiten, mit dieser Anomalie umzugehen. Während zur Zeit häufig eine altersabhängige Rationierung vorgeschlagen wird, lassen sich aus der Wirtschaftstheorie Vorschläge herleiten, die effizienter sind, wie z.B. die Entwicklung von Krankenversicherungsverträgen, die Selbstrationierung induzieren, d.h. einen etwas zurückhaltenderen Umgang mit medizinischen Innovationen gegen Ende des menschlichen Lebens fördern.

Cardiac surgery in the elderly: impact on hospital management and economics

CHAPTER **6**

M. Heberer, E. Juhasz, A. Todorov, P. Vogt, H.R. Zerkowski

■ Abstract

This paper challenges the hypothesis of limited cost-efficiency of cardiac surgery in elderly as compared to younger patients on the basis of recent data of the cardiac surgery unit of the University Hospital of Basel. A total of 1394 procedures performed in the years 1998 and 1999 was analyzed. Two hundred and fifteen patients (15.4%) were older than 75 years of age. Average age was 62.7 ± 12.1 years, LOS 12.2 ± 3.1 days, duration of intensive care 2.9 ± 3.1 days, and hospital mortality 2.2%. Neither outcome nor revenue from patients below and above age 75 were significantly different. These results are in agreement with recent reports by other groups and no longer justify numeric age limits for cardiac surgery. In consequence, the increasing proportion of the elderly population will translate into a growing demand for cardiac surgery. Appropriate actions of hospitals and health care administrations are required. We propose the following principles:

■ patient demands should be satisfied rather than rejected by rationing measures;

■ medical centres with significant case load and experience should be preferred over great numbers of service providers with limited volume. These centres provide acknowledged advantages regarding quality, cost, and innovation, particularly in areas of high-tech medicine;

■ a culture of continuous improvement pertaining to both medical and management services is a prerequisite for the aforementioned goals. In particular, the cooperation of different professional groups and medical disciplines represents a success factor for hospitals in the future. There is good evidence that actions based on these principles will enable high quality medical services for larger groups of patients at acceptable rates.

▪ Introduction

Efficacy and cost of surgery in elderly patients remain subjects of controversy based on a number of non-proven assumptions: these include the hypothesis that surgery in elderly as compared to younger patients is less effective but more costly, that outcomes are less favorable, and that society can no longer afford the economic burden as these procedures become more frequent with increasing age of the population. This paper challenges these assumptions based on data from the heart-surgery service of the University of Basel. Economic relevance for the hospital and future potential of heart surgery among other services of the University Hospital and specifically of heart surgery in the elderly was assessed. Actions that respect both the demand of patients and the economic potential of regions or nations will be proposed.

▪ Data bases and methods

Data were retrospectively derived from both the SAP data base of hospital administration and from the data base of the German Federal Task Force for Quality Management of Cardiac Diseases (Bundesarbeitsgemeinschaft Qualitätssicherung Herz). The two data bases were independent precluding joint statistical analysis.

Clinical information regarding all patients undergoing cardiac surgery in 1998 and 1999 was available from the Quality Management data base. Financial information was confined to a random sample of 30 patients drawn from the SAP data base with 15 patients below and 15 patients above 75 years of age.

Both samples were transferred to a SPSS data file (SPSS Inc., Chicago, IL) and analyzed by use of this program. Data are displayed as means and standard deviation unless specified otherwise. Differences among groups were tested by analysis of variance (AOV).

▪ The heart surgery service of the University of Basel

▪ **Patients, procedures, and outcome.** A total of 1394 cardiac procedures were performed through 1998 and 1999 in patients averaging 63.7 ± 12.1 years (median 65.6 years). The youngest patient was 3.9 years, the oldest 89.1 years. Two hundred and fifteen patients (15.4%) were beyond age 75.

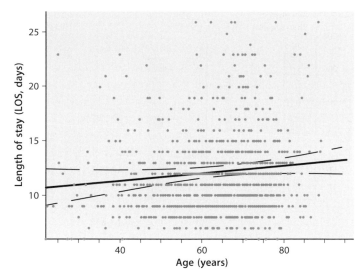

Fig. 1. Length of stay of 1394 patients who underwent heart surgery in 1998 and 1999. Linear correlation ($y = 0.96 + 0.035x$; $r = 0.055$) suggests a limited increase in LOS with age which does not attain statistical significance

Length of hospital stay (LOS) averaged 12.2 ± 8.6 days (Fig. 1), the period of care in the intensive care unit (ICU) 2.9 ± 3.1 days. Thirty patients died during hospitalization corresponding to a 2.2% hospital mortality. There was no statistically significant correlation between age and mortality.

Of the total 1394 patients 1048 (75.2%) underwent coronary artery bypass grafting (CABG) only. These patients were characterized by an average age of 65.1 ± 9.5 years, a LOS of 12.3 ± 8.8 days and an ICU stay of 2.9 ± 3.0 days. Differences between younger (<75 years: 896 patients, 86.5%) and older patients (≥75 years: 152 patients, 14.5%) regarding mortality (1.8% vs. 2.6%), ICU stay (2.9 ± 3.2 vs. 2.9 ± 1.6 days) and LOS (12.3 ± 9.4 vs. 11.8 ± 4.2 days) were not statistically significant (Fig. 2).

▪ **Economic analysis.** Cost per case was analyzed in the groups of younger (64.7 ± 7.3) and elderly patients (77.7 ± 2.5 years) who both underwent CABG only. Cost per case was $21\,580 \pm 8815$ SFR in patients of the younger and $27\,856 \pm 10\,070$ SFR in patients of the older age group. Neither this difference nor the linear regression of cost over age was statistically significant (Fig. 3).

The turnover of cardiac surgery as estimated on the basis of the 30 patients' random sample (average cost 24718 SFR) and the total number of patients operated per year (697 p.a.) amounts to 17.2 million

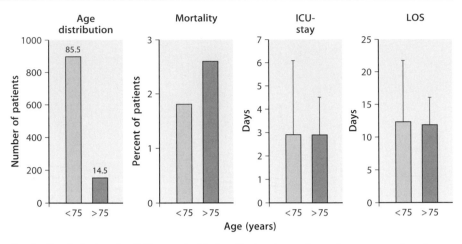

Fig. 2. Key indicators in 1048 age-stratified patients who underwent coronary artery bypass grafting (CABG) in 1998 and 1999

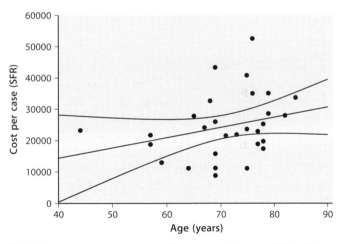

Fig. 3. Cost per case versus age. Linear correlation ($y = 1335 + 328x$; $r = 0.280$) does not attain statistical significance

SFR p.a. This value corresponds to 3.6% of the total turnover of the University Hospital of Basel (480 million SFR in 1999).

Revenues per case were found to depend primarily on the type of insurance, given the compulsory insurance coverage in Switzerland: revenues from residents of the Kanton Basel-Stadt (local patients) with only basic insurance coverage averaged 15435 ± 2356 SFR. Revenues from patients of other Kantons or from patients with supplemental insurance coverage averaged 30441 ± 5729 SFR (AOV: $p < 0.05$). In con-

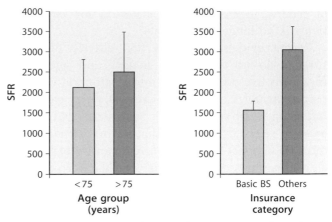

Fig. 4. Revenue structure in two groups of patients above and below 75 years of age (n = 15 each) undergoing CAPG. "basic BS" indicates coverage of residents of Basel-Stadt (local Kanton) by basic insurance; "others" summarizes all other insurance categories

trast, differences in revenues from younger (21 192 ± 6 911 SFR) and older patients undergoing heart surgery (25 068 ± 9 608 SFR) were not statistically significant (Fig. 4).

▩ Heart surgery in elderly patients

▩ **Demand and ageing.** Heart surgery can be performed with low complication rates and morbidity even in elderly patients. This represents a remarkable improvement during a comparatively short period of time. In the late sixties, an editorial of the British Medical Journal concluded that "surgical treatment for valvular disease is not at present feasible in elderly patients" [3]. Since this point in time, age limits for heart surgery have continuously been extended [16], resulting in an increase of heart procedures performed in Western countries [19].

To date, age remains one among other independent risk factors for mortality and morbidity in heart surgery, as confirmed by recent European [17] and US studies [12, 13]. The relative impact of age is comparable to many other risk factors including renal failure and reduced ejection fraction [17], suggesting that the selection of patients for heart surgery[1] should be based on physiological status as defined by a panel

---

[1] Für deutschsprachige Leser sei angemerkt, dass „selection of patients" dem Begriff der „Chirurgischen Indikation" eher entspricht als dem deutschen Verständnis von „Selektion".

of criteria. Age as a single criterion for inclusion or exclusion of patients is no longer appropriate.

Recent evidence suggests that elderly patients undergoing cardiac surgery do no worse than a sex- and age-matched population with regard to five-year survival and postoperative quality of life [1, 13]. In particular, 85% of patients over 70 years were found to be self-caring following heart surgery [13]. Such data justify heart surgery for appropriately selected elderly patients who demand the procedure. Furthermore, savings at the macro-level[2] can be expected because independent elderly patients do not require costly external assistance.

■ **Economic impact at the business level.** The contribution of heart surgery to the economic performance of the University Hospital requires careful analysis. On the one hand, heart surgery is an important business of the University Hospital: 3.6% of the total revenue of the University Hospital is generated by cardiac surgery. This contribution to the hospital revenue represents a conservative estimate because it does not take into account secondary and complex procedures that generate more revenue. Furthermore, outpatient services of cardiothoracic surgery, cardiology, and other hospital businesses that all benefit from a state-of-the-art heart surgery service are not included in this estimate.

On the other hand, the balance of average revenues and average costs amounts to a deficit of 1 588 ± 11 305 SFR per case (Fig. 4). This simplified calculation does not consider the contribution of the home Kanton to basic insurance for hospital care under the rules of recent Swiss legislation ("Neues KVG") [7]: for patients with basic insurance coverage, an equal contribution of both the insurance and the Kanton is granted. This contribution by the Kanton does not cover the hospital's deficit but represents an integrated part of Swiss hospital financing. Consideration of this contribution improves the financial statement significantly (Fig. 5).

----

[2] Die Abgrenzung von volkswirtschaftlicher („macro-level") und betriebswirtschaftlicher Sichtweise („micro-level" oder „business-level") ist für diese Betrachtung wichtig, welche den Standpunkt des Spitals analysieren soll. Grundsätzlich muss die Möglichkeit von Zielkonflikten dieser beiden Ebenen in Betracht gezogen und die Interessenidentität als (wünschenswerter) Sonderfall angesehen werden.

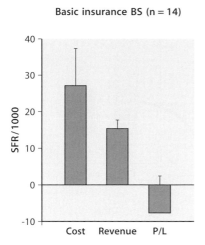 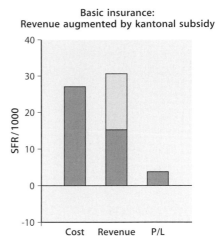

Fig. 5. Model calculation: Cost, revenue and profit/loss (P/L) for 14 residents of Basel-Stadt (BS) with basic insurance coverage undergoing CABG. P/L calculation without (left panel) and with (right panel) consideration of the statutory contribution by the Kanton Basel-Stadt (hatched area)

Furthermore, operating leverage needs to be considered when assessing the financial contribution of patients from different insurance categories[3]. This concept is based on the differentiation of fixed and variable costs. Hospitals, particularly those operating in the high-tech area of medicine, incur significant fixed costs in order to be ready for the delivery of complex services at any given point in time throughout the 365 days and nights of the year. Heart surgery requires relevant investments into complex equipment and respective maintenance, permanent availability, and continuing education of highly trained nursing staff, of expert physicians from different medical specialties (surgeons, cardiologists, anesthesiologists, others), and of technical and administrative staff. The costs of this structure can be regarded as fixed, almost irrespective of utilization. Fixed costs will surmount the variable costs incurred by each patient and procedure. Ratios between fixed and variable costs ranging between 70:30 and 80:20 appear to be both usual and acceptable. Reimbursement for surgery in patients with basic insurance coverage (without consideration of the contribution of the Kanton)

---

[3] Im deutschsprachigen Gebiet handelt es sich um die Deckungsbeitragsrechnung, welche auf der Abgrenzung von fixen und variablen Kosten beruht. Deckungsbeiträge entsprechen der Differenz zwischen am Markt erzielbaren Preisen (= Tarife) und den variablen, also direkt durch den Dienstleistungsprozess ausgelösten, Kosten. Positive Deckungsbeiträge erwirtschaften somit einen Teil der fixen Kosten einer Betriebsstruktur.

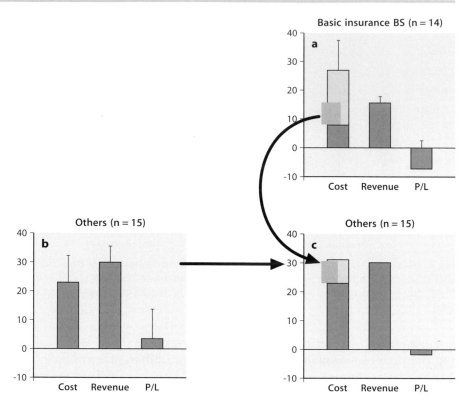

Fig. 6. Simplified P/L model illustrating the relevance of partial fixed cost coverage by contributions from basic insurance (**a**). Adding this cost (dark grey area, **a**) to the cost attributed to patients with other insurances (panel B) would turn the small profit in this patient group (**b**) into a loss (**c**). N.b. these numbers are derived from a non-representative random sample of 30 patients

will not cover all costs but clearly exceed the variable cost component. This latter part helps to finance the fixed costs of the hospital. Clearly, the hospital cannot live on the return from these cases but this contribution to the fixed costs helps financing. This contribution also decreases the charges to patients with full reimbursement: these charges would be higher without the contribution of patients with basic insurance (Fig. 6).

▪ Implications for hospital management

There is no doubt regarding the proportional increase and the growing life expectancy of the elderly population [9, 21]. The corresponding increase in the demand for cardiology and cardiac surgery services has been detailed in other chapters of this book. This development has implications for hospital management.

■ **Respect for the demands of patients.** The recent WHO report emphasizes that demands of patients rather than control of political authorities should determine the use of health care [11]: patients are responsible, informed, and sovereign. If they are not, authorities should promote responsibility, information, and sovereignty rather than patronize people.

This concept will also impact on the physician-patient relationship. Traditionally, physicians took care of their patients and were assumed to act in the best interest of their patients. Now, physicians have to deal with and treat informed patients who will demand or deny medical services on the basis of both medical and economic information. Thus, empowerment of patients – previously regarded as a part of human rights – also becomes an economic issue.

Hospital management needs to respond: we have to explore patients' needs and to provide the required services [6]. As a result, cardiac surgery will be required by and provided to an increasing number of individuals, with high quality and at acceptable cost. There is an increasing consensus that we should seek to provide this service rather than find arguments to deny required medical services, service quality, or price [6].

■ **Expert centres of medical activity.** The number of recommendations for improvement of quality and cost is countless and ever-increasing. In contrast, the number of validated measures is limited. Among those, the concepts of economy of scale, standardization, and integration of services along the value chain have stood the test of time.

The association between case load and both increasing quality and decreasing cost has been verified for a number of procedures not only in the areas of interventional cardiology [15, 18] and cardiac surgery [10, 20] but also in many other fields including general and orthopedic surgery [4, 8]. This association is no surprise in view of preceding industrial experience [2]. Thus, case load appears to translate through experience-driven process improvement, purchasing power and other factors into enhanced quality and lower cost.

Supportive effects have been shown to result from standardization and use of information technology [14]. In fact, McKinsey estimated that America's health-care bill could be cut by $250 billion a year – 25% of total expenditure – if medical organizations made an annual investment of $50 billion in information systems [5].

So, the message is in favor of large competence centres rather than decentralized clinical units of limited capacity and experience. Such centres will be able to invest in buildings, equipment, and information technology as well as in people to provide state-of-the-art services. This is obvious for high-tech areas of medicine, but most likely holds true for all other areas. Hospital strategies and organizational structures at local, regional, and national level need to correspond to these needs.

■ **Continuous improvement.** Medicine has achieved acknowledged and effective improvements of therapy. Increased performance continues to be praised; the incurred cost, however, is generally condemned. Can we find solutions to this dilemma, perhaps by learning from other industries?

Centers of medical expertise have been advocated. Much like in other industries, the efficiency of such complex businesses can be improved by integrative systems thinking rather than by further specialization of independent sub-disciplines. And this is new for medicine: we need to integrate different medical and technical specialties, different professional groups, and different service providers along the value chain (e.g., referring physicians, hospitals, rehabilitation units). The tools have been created and validated in other businesses, but they require adaptation to the medical field. Compared to others, the medical business is different particularly with regard to its ethical foundations. Correspondingly, medicine requires leadership based on expertise in both medicine and economics: economization of medicine is not in the best interests of the patient but input from economists is required to improve medical service delivery. Thus, there is no alternative to a cooperation among all professional groups that have responsibility in health care. This includes economists.

■ Conclusions

Cardiac surgery in elderly patients represents both a medical and a management model with broad implications for medicine. This field demonstrates the continuously expanding potential to treat patients, the increasing demand of patients, and the available management options to respond to these demands. The options include the formation and support for centres of medical excellence including information technology, the implementation of appropriate organizational structures with medical and economic leadership, and the integration of services along the value chain. Interprofessional and interdisciplinary cooperation within and beyond the hospital will be mandatory to appropriately serve larger groups of patients.

▪ References

1. Boucher M, Dupras A, Jutras M, Pagé V, LeLorier J, Gagnon RM (1997) Long-term survival and functional status in the elderly after cardiac surgery. Can J Cardiol 13:646–652
2. Crosby PB (1979) Quality is free. The art of making quality certain. 1. McGraw-Hill Book Company, New York
3. Editorial (1968) Systolic murmurs in the elderly. Brit Med J 530–531
4. Heberer M (1997) Qualität und Kostenreduktion: übereinstimmende Ziele einer strategischen Neuorientierung von Krankenhäusern. Langenbecks Arch Chir 382:837–839
5. Information technology (1998) Economist 71:2–28
6. Kenagy JW, Berwick DM, Shore MF (1999) Service quality in health care. JAMA 281:661–665
7. Krankenversicherung (832) (1996) Bundeskanzlei, Bern
8. Lavernia CJ, Guzman JF (1995) Relationship of surgical volume to short-term mortality, morbidity, and hospital charges in arthroplasty. J Arthroplasty 10:133–140
9. Malaguerra C (1996) Statistisches Jahrbuch der Schweiz 1997. Verlag Neue Zürcher Zeitung, Zürich, 1–464
10. Marwick C (1994) Coronary bypass grafting economics, including rehabilitation. Curr Opin Cardiol 9:635–640
11. Musgrove P, Creese A, Preker A, Baeza C, Anell A, Prentice T (2000) The World Health Report 2000. 1–206. World Health Organization, Geneva
12. Parsonnet V, Dean D, Bernstein AD (1989) A method of uniform stratification of risk for evaluating the results of surgery in acquired adult heart disease. Circulation 79:I3–I12
13. Peigh PS, Swartz MT, Vaca KJ, Lohmann DP, Naunheim KS (1994) Effect of advancing age on cost and outcome of coronary artery bypass grafting. Ann Thorac Surg 58:1362–1367
14. Pestotnik SL, Classen DC, Evans RS, Burke JP (1996) Implementing antibiotic practice guidelines through computer-assisted decision support: clinical and financial outcomes. Ann Internal Med 124:884–890
15. Phillips KA, Luft HS, Ritchie JL (1995) The association of hospital volumes of percutaneous transluminal coronary angioplasty with adverse outcomes, length of stay, and charges in California. Med Care 33:502–514
16. Reichart B, Klinner W, Kemkes BM, Kreuzer E, Peters D (1982) Koronarchirurgie im hohen Lebensalter: Indikationen und Ergebnisse. In: Heberer G, Witte J (eds) Chirurgie im hohen Alter. Perimed, Erlangen, 56–65
17. Roques F, Gabrielle F, Michel P, DeVincentiis C, David M, Baudet E (1995) Quality of care in adult heart surgery: proposal for a self-assessment approach based on a French multicenter study. Eur J Cardiothorac Surg 9:433–440

18. Shook TL, Sun GW, Burstein S, Eisenhauer AC, Matthews RV (1996) Comparison of percutaneous transluminal coronary angioplasty outcome and hospital costs for low-volume and high-volume operators. Am J Cardiol 77:331–336

19. Von Luterotti N (2000) Mehr Untersuchungen und Eingriffe am Herzen. Frankfurter Allgemeine Zeitung (260), N3. 11-8-00 Frankfurt

20. Woods JR, Saywell RM Jr, Nyhuis AW, Jay SJ, Lohrman RG, Halbrook HG (1992) The learning curve and the cost of heart transplantation. Health Serv Res 27:219–238

21. Zweifel P, Felder S, Meier M (1996) Demographische Alterung und Gesundheitskosten: eine Fehlinterpretation. In: Oberender P (ed) Alter und Gesundheit. Nomos Verlagsgesellschaft, Baden-Baden, 29–46

◾ Herzchirurgische Eingriffe bei Älteren – Bedeutung für das Krankenhaus-Management und wirtschaftliche Faktoren

M. Heberer, E. Juhasz, A. Todorov, P. Vogt, H. R. Zerkowski

Diese Arbeit stellt die Hypothese der begrenzten Kosteneffektivität herzchirurgischer Eingriffe bei älteren im Vergleich zu jüngeren Patienten in Frage. Die Grundlage dafür sind neuere Ergebnisse der herzchirurgischen Abteilung der Universitätsklinik Basel. Es wurden insgesamt 1394 Eingriffe aus den Jahren 1998 und 1999 ausgewertet. 215 Patienten (15,4%) waren älter als 75 Jahre. Das Durchschnittsalter betrug 62,7 ± 12,1 Jahre, die Dauer des Klinikaufenthalts 12,2 ± 3,1 Tage, die Aufenthaltsdauer auf der Intensivstation 2,9 ± 3,1 Tage und die Mortalität während des Klinikaufenthalts 2,2%. Weder der Behandlungserfolg noch die Einkünfte zeigten bei Patienten oberhalb und unterhalb von 75 Jahren signifikante Unterschiede. Diese Ergebnisse stimmen mit Berichten anderer Gruppen überein, sodass Altersgrenzen für herzchirurgische Eingriffe nach dem kalendarischen Alter nicht mehr gerechtfertigt sind. Daraus folgt, dass sich der wachsende Anteil der älteren Bevölkerung in einer wachsenden Nachfrage nach herzchirurgischen Eingriffen niederschlagen wird und dass Krankenhäuser und Einrichtungen der Gesundheitsvorsorge adäquate Maßnahmen ergreifen müssen. Als Grundsätze schlagen wir vor:

- ◾ Die Nachfrage der Patienten sollte befriedigt werden, anstatt sie durch Rationierungsmaßnahmen zurückzuweisen.
- ◾ Medizinischen Zentren mit hoher Fallzahl und großer Erfahrung ist gegenüber einer großen Zahl von Anbietern mit begrenzter Kapazität der Vorzug zu geben. Diese Zentren bieten im Hinblick auf Qualität, Kosten und Innovationen anerkannte Vorteile, und zwar insbesondere in Bereichen der hochtechnologisierten Medizin.
- ◾ Voraussetzung für die genannten Ziele ist eine Kultur der ständigen Verbesserung sowohl der medizinischen Leistungen als auch des Managements. In Zukunft stellt insbesondere die Zusammenarbeit unterschiedlicher Berufsgruppen und medizinischer Fachgebiete einen Erfolgsfaktor für Krankenhäuser dar. – Es gibt ausreichend Anhaltspunkte dafür, dass ein auf diesen Grundsätzen basierendes Vorgehen qualitativ hochwertige medizinische Leistungen für größere Patientengruppen und zu akzeptablem Preis ermöglichen wird.

CHAPTER 7 Viewpoint of a Swiss health insurer

A. RYCHEN

■ Comments on the public view of in-patient treatment of cardiovascular diseases

An example from the canton of Zurich: The cardiac surgery and cardiology clinics of a well-known hospital centre opened their doors to the public. That very morning hundreds of visitors passed along the corridors with their exhibition walls. They sought out the cardiac catheterisation laboratory and looked over the instruments and apparatuses used in cardiology examinations and in heart operations, laid out in rows. Open heart surgery could be seen on video. They were introduced to modern non-invasive uses and diagnoses. The hospital focuses on rapid, uncomplicated but nevertheless thorough examination methods. The American Chest Brain Centres serve as a reference. The necessary attention is paid to the treatment chain and the functional demarcation with the nearby university hospital.

This substantial public interest precludes any further doubt: The heart – in this medical sense of the term as well – rules our insurees. Certainly most is known about the risk factors of cardiovascular diseases. But can I avoid them, stress for example and smoking, and do I want to? And if disease sets in, possibly despite all that, what can I expect, to what hopes do medical science and its high technology instrumentarium give rise? The clinical interest of the elderly visitors also, encouraged by the imminent threat and the simultaneous hope that medical science will be able to put a large amount right again.

■ Further preliminary remarks

The organisers of this meeting are now asking for the point of view of a Swiss health insurer on the problems of heart diseases in old age.

First of all on the subject of *age*: I represent a health insurer who follows the law on social health insurance to the letter; in other words according to the so-called principle of mutuality which excludes the unequal treatment of insured parties. Senior citizens are not a peripheral, marginal or even marginisable group; this is already prohibited by the social generation contract. They represent 15% of the total population today and this proportion will continue to increase. The number has more than doubled since 1950 and among over-80-year olds it has quadrupled. The fact that health service costs tend to increase with advancing age and reach their pinnacle in the final year of life is well known. Their redistribution is a touchstone of the solidarity between generations. I am able to say this as the chairman of Visana with the prospect of some credibility. In basic insurance, however, complete equality of treatment applies today from the age of 25 years onwards in respect of premiums, cost sharing and claims to services.

On the subject of *heart diseases in age*: Improved living conditions and successful medical treatments have increased the average life expectancy (men 76, women 82). This however also means that diseases continue today up to an advanced age, occasionally accentuated and as such incurring costs. However, the number of years gained in good health is frequently cited as an indicator of the growing effectiveness of the health system. Who would not fundamentally welcome this development; the health insurance funds possibly, as agents of their insurees and trustees of social security resources? Are not these heart diseases which nowadays can occur up to an advanced age precisely the expression of these improved medical possibilities which you as doctors can provide your patients and our insurees?

On the subject of the basic attitude of the *health insurers*: It is known that health insurers assume the cost risks of their insurees against payment of premiums and that they offset these within the risk community. The insurees give their insurers a mandate: to fund the costs of illness against payment of a premium or to make good the associated loss of income. This task of redistribution has been assumed traditionally by the health insurance funds and the term "fund" provides the correct impression that the outflows of money must be offset by sufficient inflows because otherwise, as is universally known, this results in an inability to pay.

The costs incurred by the health insurers have grown dramatically in the last decades. In their capacity as premium and tax payers, our insurees suffer from a financial burden which they pay as recipients of a service. There are constantly pressing demands (with which the representatives of the economic sciences and the authorities concur) for the "funds," finally and at their earliest convenience, to adopt an active approach and to ensure that the costs of medical service provision, and also their own internal costs, are reduced. It is therefore a matter of looking closely at hospitals, doctors, etc. and where necessary rapping their knuckles. Since then health insurers and their associations have fought for a limitation of resources, better tariffs and for a limitation of the increase in quantity while maintaining the quality of the result. Often therefore health insurers find themselves wrongly suspected by their insurees of wanting to ration where they are simply seeking an acceptable level of costs. It is however necessary to point out here that expectations placed on the insurers in this respect quite simply cannot be met. The jurisdiction and resources allocated to them by the legislator simply do not suffice.

▪ Some data and facts

When one speaks as a non-medic and non-cardiologist at a specialist event like yours here, the mention of data and facts can easily be viewed as a tiresome repetition of what has already been said and is already known. I shall therefore confine myself to the following graphs (Figs. 1–7).

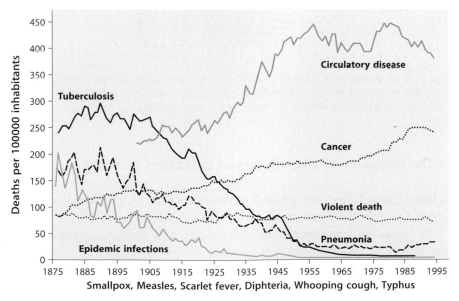

Fig. 1. Main causes of death in the last 120 years (source: Federal Office of Statistics). In Switzerland, cardiovascular diseases are the leading cause of death. Fortunately, between 1980 and 1997 a 9% decline was observed

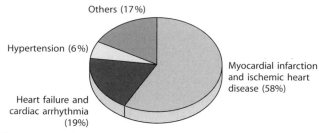

Fig. 2. Heart diseases as a cause of death in 1997 by type (source: Pharma-Information). In 1997 about three-quarters of deaths from cardiovascular diseases were due to heart disease. The predominant causes of death here were myocardial infarction and other ischaemic heart diseases

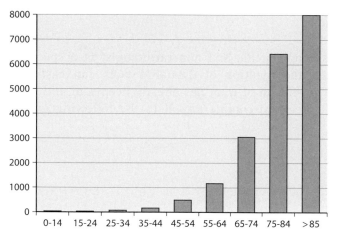

Fig. 3. Heart diseases as a cause of death in 1994 by age (source: Federal Institute of Statistics). The number of deaths as a result of heart diseases increases exponentially with age. Long-term comparisons show that life expectancy in heart patients has also increased substantially

■ The viewpoint of a health insurer in matters of detail

I have showed that the general economic costs of cardiovascular diseases, but also the direct costs, are considerable, particularly in old age.

In respect of cost limitation, affordability and quality, I have come to the following conclusions:

■ In my understanding, the risk factors of cardiovascular diseases have now been extensively investigated. The factors of poor nutrition, smoking, lack of exercise and stress have been recognised as being at least in part amenable to change. This knowledge should be used in preventive medicine and communicated extensively to the population

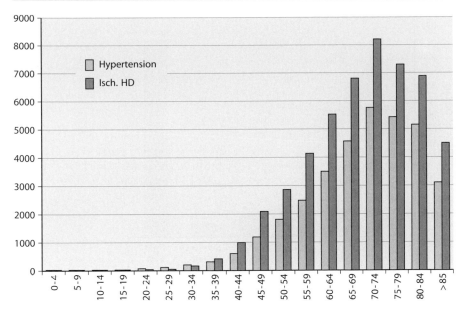

Fig. 4. Hypertension and ischemic heart disease, number of diagnoses by age (source: "Global" medical statistics of Swiss hospitals 1995). The previous figure is highly correlated with the statistics on medical diagnoses in hospitals represented here. The need for inpatient treatment is showing a tendency to increase, as in other specialist medical areas, with the patient's age

of all age groups. The earlier one starts with this, the better the pro-

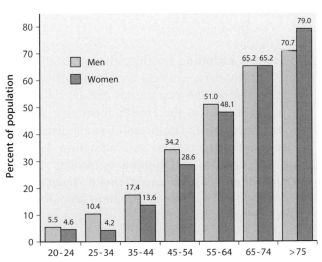

Fig. 5. Estimated prevalence of cardiovascular diseases in Americans, USA, 1988–1994, by age and sex (source: American Heart Association). This American graph confirms the previous picture for Switzerland

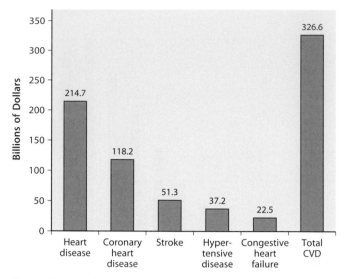

Fig. 6. Estimated direct and indirect costs of cardiovascular diseases and stroke, USA 2000 (American Heart Association). The right-hand column depicts the aggregate estimated direct and indirect costs in the current year (because of overlaps, the five left-hand columns cannot simply be added together). It is divided as follows: of the 327 000 million dollars, $ 186 000 million are direct costs, of which 70% are incurred by hospitals, 15% by doctors and other medical personnel, 9% by drugs and 6% homes and rehabilitation centres. The indirect costs from lost productivity are estimated as $ 141 000 million: one-fifth from morbidity, four-fifths from mortality. In Switzerland, Sagmeister and others estimated the costs of ischaemic heart disease alone for 1993 as 2 100 million SFR., of which about 1,000 million SFR. were direct costs

spects are, including for the elderly.

Service providers, insurers and authorities should not tire in their efforts to inform the population constantly and repeatedly about these facts. As is known, the Health Insurance Act quite specifically in Article 19 prescribes the promotion of disease prevention. The consequence was the creation of Foundation 19 which is operated jointly with the cantons and funded by money from our insurees. It must stimulate, co-ordinate and evaluate "measures to promote health and prevent diseases". I mention here also the Swiss Heart Foundation which in my opinion provides excellent information and offers an exemplary model for our enterprise in its method of operation. (Visana Versicherungen itself has a foundation for health promotion and prevention. With at present still very modest means, it encourages projects of this kind. As distinct from the Heart Foundation, however, it is not centred on one specific body).

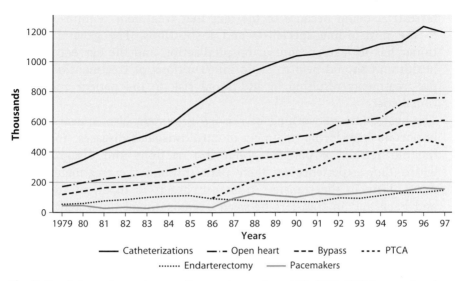

Fig. 7. Trends in cardiovascular operations and procedures, USA, 1979–1997 (source: American Heart Association). This graph, lastly, depicts trends in the use of invasive operations. These offer hope to many patients and the belief in a second or third chance, which is also increasingly being fulfilled as procedures continue to improve. In addition, they naturally generate massive direct costs

▩ I consider the early detection of risk factors in medical practice and the systematic persuasion and involvement of patients in terms of the necessary changes of behaviour to be very important, not least for cost reasons. It is specifically the general practitioner who plays a central role in detecting emergent risk factors and in secondary prevention. In the health survey of 1997, the answers of many of those questioned showed a considerable degree of uncertainty as to whether and when they had last had their cholesterol levels and high blood pressure measured. The general practitioner is not exposed to the accusation of pursuing private monetary interests if he were to arrange such examinations at suitable intervals and call in or invite his patients to these as necessary. If further proof is needed of this, then most recently the WHO's Monica Project has convincingly demonstrated the close relationship between risk factors and heart diseases.

▩ In addition, I would like to see a systematic networking of general practitioners with cardiologists, heart clinics and follow-up care institutions. General practitioners should, and often want to, continue to follow and care for their cardiac patients in their progress through the treatment chain. The cardiac patient does not become an extraterrestrial being because of the fact that treatment requires referral to the next-in-line specialists and institutions. The general practitioner has to take account of hospitalisation and the current state of health and should help to avoid interruptions of treatment or multiple treatments resulting in additional risk to the patient and additional cost.

■ The systematic networking of service providers also appears to me important here in the treatment of cardiovascular diseases. You know the old refrain of patients about the frictions and disagreements which they experience on their path through the treatment chain, particularly in the transfers from outpatient to inpatient treatment and back and in transfers between organisational units and institutions. In the last few years in particular, including in the canton of Bern where we have our head office, major efforts at coordination have been undertaken. The health insurers welcome this progress from the points of view of quality and cost and hope that this procedure will become even more systematic.

■ Today we are faced with an admirable state of the art in the medical treatment and follow-up of cardiovascular diseases. And if all else fails, cardiac patients, and particularly the elderly, can profit from a wide range of high-tech invasive interventions. These options are the results of medical research, the expression of high medical knowledge and skills and not in any way a matter of course. A country which has also opened up these possibilities for itself must have considerable prosperity, for these operations are expensive. In this context we demand that, as is provided for in Art. 58 KVG, the service providers who are permitted to undertake the particularly expensive or difficult examinations or treatments at the expense of the basic insurance should be more closely identified. KVG Art. 43 Section 2 Letter d points in the same direction. Quality dictates and cost efficiency constitute the impetus to these conditions.

■ Moreover I set great store by the possibilities of the new statistics. The introduction in particular of a uniform tariff structure for individual services valid for the whole of Switzerland will, by virtue of the binding nomenclature, allow evaluations that show which service provider provides which medical measures to what extent, at what costs and for which patients. They will provide appropriate bases for assessment and show where statistically relevant deviations occur. They will also provide hard data for the topic discussed today. In the same way the new administrative and medical statistics from the hospitals, in which the Federal Office for Statistics is achieving good progress according to reports, point in the same direction.

▪ Today the database is still modest. Our attempts to highlight the cost consequences of heart diseases and the involvement of the older section of the population in them are almost embarrassingly rudimentary. For precisely this reason the opinion of the insurers is shared by many specialists among the service providers: that there are still considerable possibilities for increased efficiencies in terms of the extent and allocation of resources, in the distinction between central, regional and peripheral functions and in the improved management of the treatment pathway through outpatient and inpatient units.

How much should be spent on the health system is the result of a pan-social consensus. Nowadays it is about 40 000 million Francs. But common sense and the law require that the resources invested should be used economically, effectively and efficiently. Four years ago a senior fund representative described 20 to 25% of the Swiss healthcare system as "air which we can expel without suffering any loss of quality". This also still needs to be confirmed by reliable data. The statement however leads me on to my last point:

▪ The search for increased efficiency and rationalisation must precede any kind of rationing measures at all costs. Rationing from our point of view is the last resort. At this meeting which deals with cardiovascular diseases *in old age*, I would draw attention specifically to the fact that I am not in any way or sense advocating specific rationing of health services to elderly persons.

I know that you are faced with precisely the same questions in heart transplantations in view of the limited number of donor organs and you must decide on the basis of recognised criteria. In my opinion a general, socially accepted agreement should in the meanwhile be sought as to the conditions under which rationing should or must at some point be introduced at all into the health system and utilised.

How much is health actually worth to us. Ethically, morally, humanly and above all when it involves ourselves or our dearest, should medicine engender apparently unlimited costs?

This deliberately provocative statement should, in contrast to the universally apparent opposition to ever higher taxes and premiums, lead us on to the vitally necessary discussion about the limitations in the health system that may possibly become necessary. This debate cannot be delegated either to the medical profession or to science or to the politicians. It is the duty of the whole of society to ask these questions. People in the so-called modern and post-modern world can also probably not avoid considering their relationship with life and death. It will be a highly challenging task to find generally acceptable criteria for universal rationing.

Personally I agree with the view that the objective degree of suffering and the foreseeable success of treatment are the main criteria for the decision and not the age that has been reached.

Sichtweise eines Schweizer Krankenversicherers

A. Rychen

Vorbemerkungen. Wenn nach der Sichtweise eines Schweizer Krankenversicherers zur Problematik der Herzkrankheiten im Alter gefragt wird, so erfordert die eigentliche Antwort drei Vorbemerkungen:

- Zum *Alter:* Die Visana führt die soziale Krankenversicherung nach dem Buchstaben des Gesetzes durch, d.h. gemäss dem Grundsatz der Gegenseitigkeit, der eine Ungleichbehandlung der Versicherten ausschliesst. Senioren sind für sie keine auszugrenzende Gruppe. Dass die Kosten mit wachsendem Alter tendenziell zunehmen und im letzten Lebensjahr ihren Kulminationspunkt finden, ist bekannt. Ihre Umverteilung ist ein Prüfstein für die Solidarität zwischen den Generationen. Heute gilt in der Grundversicherung völlige Gleichbehandlung bezüglich Prämien, Kostenbeteiligungen und Leistungsansprüchen.

- Zu den *Herzkrankheiten im Alter:* Als Indikator für wachsende Effektivität des Gesundheitswesens wird häufig die Zahl gewonnener Lebensjahre bei guter Gesundheit herangezogen. Wer möchte diese Entwicklung grundsätzlich nicht begrüssen, die Krankenkassen etwa, als Mandanten ihrer Versicherten und Treuhänder von Sozialversicherungsgeldern? Sind diese Heart Diseases, die nun bis ins hohe Alter auftreten können, nicht gerade Ausdruck dieser verbesserten medizinischen Möglichkeiten, die die Ärzte ihren Patienten bzw. unseren Versicherten zukommen lassen?

- Zu den *Kosten:* Die Krankenversicherer und ihre Verbände kämpfen um eine Beschränkung der Ressourcen, bessere Tarife, für eine Limitierung des Mengenwachstums bei Beibehaltung der Ergebnisqualität. Die Versicherten nehmen zu dieser Tätigkeit eine etwas zwiespältige Haltung ein: Als Prämien- und Steuerzahler fordern sie sie, als Leistungsbezieher ist sie ihnen beinahe lästig.

Zur Sichtweise eines Krankenversicherers im Einzelnen: Die volkswirtschaftlichen, aber auch die direkten Kosten von Herz-Kreislaufkrankheiten sind, besonders in höherem Alter, erheblich.

Mit dem Blick auf Kostenbegrenzung sowie Finanzierbarkeit und Qualität gilt folgendes:

- Die Risikofaktoren der Herzkreislaufkrankheiten sind heute weitgehend erforscht. Als mindestens teilweise beeinflussbar gelten die Faktoren falsche Ernährung, Rauchen, Bewegungsmangel und Stress. Dieses Wissen ist präventivmedizinisch zu nutzen und der Bevölkerung aller Altersklassen eingehend zu kommunizieren.

■ Die Früherkennung der Risikofaktoren in der Arztpraxis sowie die systematische Beeinflussung und der Einbezug des Patienten im Hinblick auf Verhaltensänderungen sind wichtig. Gerade der Hausarzt/ die Hausärztin spielt bei der Erhebung von aufgetretenen Risikofaktoren und bei der sekundären Prävention eine zentrale Rolle.

■ Der Referent würde sich eine systematische Vernetzung der Hausärzte mit den Kardiologen, den Herzkliniken und Nachsorgeinstitutionen wünschen. Es soll vermieden werden, dass Behandlungsunterbrüche bzw. Mehrfachbehandlungen zu zusätzlichem Risiko für den Patienten und zu zusätzlichen Kosten führen.

■ Heute blickt man auf einen bewundernswerten State of the Art in der medizinischen Behandlung und Nachbehandlung von Herzkreislaufkrankheiten. Und wenn alle Stricke reissen, so können am Herzen erkrankte Personen, und zwar ganz besonders auch ältere Personen, von einer reichen Palette invasiver Hightechinterventionen profitieren. Die hierfür berechtigten Leistungserbringer sind näher zu bezeichnen (cf. Art. 58 KVG).

■ Grosse Hoffnung wird in die Möglichkeiten der neuen Statistik gesetzt. Gerade die Einführung einer gesamtschweizerisch gültigen einheitlichen Tarifstruktur für Einzelleistungen wird wegen der verbindlichen Nomenklatur Auswertungen gestatten, die aufzeigen, welche Leistungserbringer welche medizinischen Massnahmen in welchem Umfang, zu welchen Kosten und für welche Patienten erbringen. Diese werden sachgerechte Beurteilungsgrundlagen zeitigen und zeigen, wo statistisch relevante Abweichungen vorkommen. Sie werden auch zum heute diskutierten Thema harte Daten bringen.

■ Es ist Ergebnis eines gesamtgesellschaftlichen Konsenses, wieviel für das Gesundheitswesen ausgegeben werden soll. Heute sind es rund 40 Mrd. Franken. Aber der gesunde Menschenverstand und das Gesetz verlangen, dass die eingesetzten Mittel wirtschaftlich, wirksam und zweckmässig eingesetzt werden.

■ Suche nach erhöhter Effizienz und Rationalisierung haben allfälligen Rationierungsmassnahmen auf jeden Fall voranzugehen. Rationierung ist aus unserer Sicht die ultima ratio. An diesem Kongress, der sich mit Herzkreislaufkrankheiten *im Alter* befasst, weist der Referent ausdrücklich darauf hin, dass er mit keinem Wort und mit keinem Gedanken eine gezielte Rationierung von Gesundheitsleistungen bei älteren Personen propagiert. Es ist eine generelle, gesellschaftlich akzeptierte Übereinkunft anzustreben, unter welchen Bedingungen Rationierung im Gesundheitswesen dereinst überhaupt eingeführt und angewendet werden darf oder muss. Der Mensch der so genannten Moderne und Postmoderne kommt dabei wohl auch nicht umhin, sein Verhältnis zu Leben und Tod zu überdenken. Es wird höchst anspruchsvoll sein, allgemein akzeptable Kriterien für eine allfällige Rationierung zu finden. Das objektivierte Mass des Leidens und des voraussichtlichen Heilungserfolges müssten dabei die wichtigsten Kriterien für den Entscheid sein und nicht das bereits erreichte Alter.

CHAPTER 8

Rationalisation or rationing – ways out of the ever increasing dilemma?

G. ZISSELSBERGER

■ Status Quo

Cost situation

In Germany, the sectors of outpatient treatment and inpatient treatment are strictly segregated. There are admittedly demands from all sides to recognise integrated care as a possible provisional solution to the problems, but in my opinion the outpatient/inpatient interlinking is far from being as successful as this would require, i.e. there are insufficient incentives to transfer services between sectors. The hospital is forced for budgetary reasons to retain as far as possible all the services it provided previously, even if these could long ago have been provided on an outpatient basis. The outpatient area does not receive sufficient financial incentives to want to provide services from the inpatient sector in an ambulatory form.

This results in part in "grotesque situations". Hospital managers are obliged to tie themselves in knots, doctors must deal more with budgetary matters than they would like. Naturally I am not talking about hospitals in this area, but far-distant regions.

The costs for a bypass operation (case-based lump sum 09021) are 24 405 DM. Naturally there are additional costs such as the basic care rate or the cardiology departmental care rate, but that is not relevant to this context.

The costs for the operation of a valvular heart disease (case-based lump sum 09091) are at present 28 756.67 DM. What has just been said applies here also.

Agreement on the number of operations in a hospital's budget

At this point I do not want to trouble you with budgetary questions and explanations, other than to say the following:

The insurance funds and the hospitals in Germany agree prospectively on a budget, i.e. the number of bypass operations is agreed. If that number is not reached, the hospitals receive a compensation payment. If the number is exceeded, the hospital does not receive the full amounts, but only a part. In this way policy is intended to emphasise the responsibility of the hospitals and where possible achieve precision landings.

■ **Conclusion.** If the observer were to interpret this in the strictest sense, he would come to the conclusion that the agreement on operations already represents a certain rationing. I cannot agree with this for the following reason:

The chairman of the German medical association referred to 50000 knee operations undertaken unnecessarily last year in Germany. I thus consider the agreement on the number of operations not as rationing but as a necessary safeguard to ensure that in fact only those people are operated upon who actual require this surgery.

Moreover, it appears not just to be a problem in Germany, because our colleague Mr Becker from the Caisse Primaire in Mühlhausen has reported a survey in the Strasbourg region in which 1000 appendix operations were assessed. The outcome was that 30% of the operations were not necessary at all.

■ Political targets

The federal government has set itself the target of reducing incidental labour costs to less than 40%. This is a very ambitious target and associated with all sorts of hurdles.

The achievement of this target at the end of the legislative period is dependent on the resolution of the reform congestion in the areas of tax, pension insurance, unemployment insurance and health insurance. How difficult this conversion is can be seen from the debates on the tax and pension reform. Solutions are in sight in the case of pension insurance for maintaining the contribution rate in the long run at the lower level that has now been achieved.

In health insurance, however, things do not look good. In order to achieve the overall target, the average contribution rate in Germany must be less than 13.0%. At present it is 13.5%, which would still be acceptable. However violent storm clouds are gathering on the horizon which would not cause a reduction in health fund contributions but quite the opposite.

■ **Conclusion.** The political targets are understandable because only with low incidental labour costs will the problem of unemployment become easier to resolve. The federal government however has serious problems in reaching its ambitious target. For health insurance, this target will not be achievable by the end of the legislative period with the "mini-reform" to date.

■ Situation of the health insurance funds

Income side

■ **Imminent income shortfalls.** The legal health insurance system is shortly to be confronted with a highly problematical development in terms of financing in the years 2001/2002. The optimistic estimate of the federal government on the publication of the SHI (Statutory Health Insurance) finance data for the first half of 2000 cannot be shared. This is due to the following reasons in particular, which in the future will entail burdens upon the SHI:

1. Ruling of the Federal Constitution Court
on contribution payment by pensioners
The ruling is in principle to be welcomed since the previous unequal treatment in the health insurance contributions of pensioners has resulted in the fact that voluntarily insured pensioners had in some cases on reaching pensionable age suddenly to pay relatively much higher contributions than during their working life. At present it is not yet possible to foresee which specific changes in the law, required by the Federal Constitution Court by 31 March 2002, will result from the ruling. According to rough calculations, simply transferring the currently applicable legal situation of compulsorily insured pensioners to voluntarily insured pensioners – a possibility for the new legal regulation put forward by the Federal Constitution Court – will result in a loss of income for the global SHI system of 500 million DM annually.

2. Ruling of the Federal Constitution Court on one-off payments
In its decision, the Federal Constitution Court comes to the conclusion that it is an infringement of the general principle of equality if contributions are taken from one-off payments without these being taken into account in wage replacement benefits (e.g. sickness benefit). The legislator was instructed to undertake the necessary legal clarifications by 30 June 2001.

It is to be feared that on the basis of the public pressure from the media, unions, patient associations, etc. a retrospective regulation – and hence extremely financially burdensome on the SHI – must be concluded.

3. Reduction in fund contributions of unemployment benefit recipients

In the current state of knowledge, there will be a further reduction in the contribution assessment basis for unemployment benefit recipients. Already as a result of the pension reform that entered into effect at the beginning of the 1990s, the SHI has been burdened by the fact that the health fund contributions for the unemployed were reduced to 80%. Now the situation is that only 58% of the final gross wage is to constitute the basis of the contribution payment for unemployment benefit recipients, not 80% as before. An extra burden on the SHI in the sum of 1 200 million DM from the year 2001 has been calculated.

4. Pension reform 2001

The planned pension reform will result in lower contribution income for the health funds from two points of view. In the first place there is a relationship between the exemption from taxes for preventive care expenditure and the exemption from contributions in social insurance. Secondly there will be lower contribution income as a result of the successive reductions in the basic pension level from the present 70% of the mean net income.

5. Pan-German risk structure compensation scheme (RSCS)

The pan-German RSCS to be introduced gradually from the year 2001 will burden the West German insurance funds with increased contribution rates of on average up to 0.4 percentage points. The financial flows from the west will place the East German funds in the position of being able to charge more favourable contribution rates than the western funds or will raise desires among service providers in the East to obtain higher reimbursements through these financial transfers. In this way the desired effects of a reduction in contribution premium in the East that is being sought would fall flat and overall the contribution rate level in Germany would increase considerably.

Increases in contribution rates in the western funds in addition will be associated with considerable competitive disadvantages for many funds because insurees have a special right of cancellation following an increase in contribution rate. If western funds are unable to keep their contribution rates stable because of their reciprocal arrangements, they are threatened with additional losses of members because an increase in contribution rate justifies immediate cancellation. In this way a vicious downward spiral would develop because the migrations will open up new financial gaps which again can only be covered by increases in contribution rates.

6. Competitive distortions
through virtual company health insurance funds (CHIF)

So-called virtual company health insurance funds which exclusively insure young and healthy members on the basis of careful risk selection are driving the legal funds, such as the local health care funds, Barmen, DAK or traditional company and guilds' health insurance funds which bear the costs of the provision of services, into a dangerous situation. According to all our analyses, the insurees leaving the provider funds were almost exclusively those who had not been serious ill in the last few years before changing their fund. Simply for the local health care funds, the resultant loss of contribution cover since the introduction of freedom of choice has amounted to about 1000 million DM. These contributions can also not be recouped by improved cost and provision management. Under the current framework conditions, it is not competition for cheaper provision that is rewarded but brutal risk selection. In this case only a fast-acting organisational reform can help. Any delay or even a postponement to the next legislative period will produce a situation which policy will no longer be possible to overturn.

Effects on contribution rate stability and incidental labour costs

A financial shortfall of about 1 800 million DM is assumed for the SHI for the year 2000. In 2001 this already deficient financial position will worsen still further as a result of the implementation of the full financial effectiveness of the additional SHI burdens mentioned.

The SHI deficit to be covered in 2001 will in all likelihood amount to 5000 million DM, or about 0.3 contribution rate points. As a consequence, an increase in the contribution rates in the year 2001 of this order of magnitude of about 14% is threatened across the whole of Germany. The provision funds in particular, which provide comprehensive cover for patients' health and medical care, will have to increase their contribution rates substantially.

▪ **Conclusion.** Despite the reduction in the contribution rate in the pension insurance, there will be no reduction in incidental labour costs. This is because in the SHI the contribution rates will increase. The target laid down in the coalition contract of 20.10.1998 for the legislative period to 2002 of a reduction in social insurance contributions to less than 40% of the net wage will therefore be missed.

Are improvements possible?

Yes, if one reverses all these things. This demand however is very unlikely to be met. For this reason we must therefore all assume that against the background of these poor framework conditions the avoidance of increases in contribution rates will only be possible for those funds which apply to themselves precisely those rationalisation restrictions that they require of their contract partners. Here too therefore innovation will be required.

The health insurance funds (and hence self-administration) must in the very short-term be given scope to become more flexible in establishing contracts with the contract partners.

Expenditure side

▪ **Imminent increases in expenditure.** I should like to confine myself to two factors, namely the shift within the age pyramid and the progress of medicine. These two things alone will result in increases in expenditure. The progress of medicine – and this I do not need to explain to you – is desirable/necessary and like many other things has assumed a breakneck speed. In most cases this costs money.

▪ **Counter-control measures.** The most successful counter-control measures would be to prevent ageing and to hold up progress. This however does not appear particularly sensible or realistic to my mind. Perhaps also as a result of the decoding of genes we might reach a state in which somehow the ageing process is brought under control. But a lot of water will still flow under the bridge before then and we must concern ourselves with the current and realistic situation.

Counter-control measures can only come from ourselves. What do I mean by this? Emergency situations have always had the positive corollary that they have given rise to innovations. In all areas there are unbelievable possibilities of rationalisation and we must manage to put these into practice. Perhaps a small example from the outpatient area: The idea of practice networks is taking physical shape. We in Lörrach have very good prospects of concluding an agreement shortly with such a network and starting it up.

Further counter-control measures involve economic reserves and overcapacities. It is not so long ago that the existence of economic reserves in the German health system was vehemently disputed. The Federal German hospitals were squeezed "like a lemon", drug budgets were calculated too low and outpatient medical care was faced with collapse because of inadequate fees. "More money in the system" at the time was the slogan of one part of Federal policy.

However in the meanwhile the health policy wind has turned. High time too. In my opinion there are considerable economic reserves. In practical terms false incentives result in an almost wasteful use of short resources in all areas of provision of the SHI: duplicate examinations, extensive use of apparatuses, a large number of avoidable hospitalisations/operations and a relatively long hospitalisation period in international terms are only some of the indicators of how much air is still present in the Federal German health system.

In addition there are overcapacities in almost all areas, whether pharmacists, hospital beds or panel doctor places. It is almost already a truism to my mind in health economics that a high density of physicians causes health expenditure to increase disproportionately.

▦ **Conclusion.** The income side of the legal health insurance system is being further undermined. The expenditure side however will continue to grow despite budgeting. The employment of economic reserves through rationalisation and the dismantling of overcapacities can close the ever widening gap between income and expenditure, at least for a certain time.

▦ Future of the health system

Targeting of services

A further subject which in future must be discussed to a greater extent involves the list of services of the legal health insurance system. This is not for me a matter of discussing a basic or a voluntary provision model or the division of the list into statutory and additional services. That is quite a different matter. The basic idea is that the service currently on offer should be provided in a more targeted way to those in need.

At the end, the opinion of the Federal committee of doctors and health funds must be further bolstered to issue prescription guidelines. For the area of medical devices it is conceivable that the doctor can no longer prescribe a specific medical device but that the exact form of the prescription should be placed in the hands of specialists within the health funds. Further potential could be achieved in the area of drugs through guidelines from the Federal Committee.

Economic reserves through new information technology

The future of the health system is to a large extent characterised by new technologies and their responsible use. For this reason, for example, the Baden-Württemberg local health insurance fund has taken over the management of the health system for the area as part of the initiative D21 set up by the Federal government. This is an example of optimised communication channels between doctors and one another, but also with patients and health funds, by which economic reserves can be mobilised which are urgently needed in the health system.

I should like here to offer another catchword: the extension of the chip card in terms of a patient identity card with medical data. Thus, at present for example the health insurance card is merely a proof of membership which is produced at considerable expense and whose use is relatively minimal. Consideration should be given as to whether this chip card could not also be used to store emergency data. In the same way, however, information could also be stored on the card by the attending physician in terms of an electronic prescription. The transmission of the prescription by internet to a pharmacist specified by the patient is thus possible without problem, i.e. transactions can be arranged very much more efficiently.

In addition, an extensive network of different partners of the health system is created. Unfortunately numerous barriers – particularly of a data protection nature – prevent a meaningful use. Initiative D21 will make its contribution to this so that similar restrictive obstructions can be eliminated to the benefit of the insured patients.

By means of so-called health portals in the internet, due allowance can be made for the great interest on the part of the population in consultation and information.

This list can be continued ad infinitum. This shows the speed at which the health system is catching up with the progress in information technology. The potential savings which are possible as a result are there for the taking. Assuming we could save only 1% of our total expenditure, we would be talking about a sum of the order of 2 500 million DM. That is a sum of money which no health reform could achieve so rapidly in terms of potential savings.

Changes through the introduction of DRGs

From 2004 DRGs are to be introduced here on the model of the Australian system. The hospital side and the health funds have agreed in principle one day before the expiry of the deadline.

At the moment things are progressing and being assessed on both sides. Certainly the question will also be raised as who will benefit most from which regulation. In principle, however, at least I believe so, the following conclusion can already be drawn: With the introduction of DRGs, those hospitals that work to high levels of quality and with an economic bias will be rewarded.

▪ Conclusion

- ▪ Rationalisation is possible.
- ▪ Rationing is not the necessary consequence.
- ▪ There is sufficient potential to be able to close the widening gap between income and expenditure, admittedly not in the long-term, but for a certain time.
- ▪ The correct financial incentives must be created.
- ▪ A health reform in Germany is urgently necessary.

■ Rationalisierung oder Rationierung –
Wege aus dem immer größer werdenden Dilemma?

G. Zisselsberger

Die Kostensituation in Deutschland stellt sich, ganz vereinfacht ausgedrückt, so dar, dass die Einnahme- und Ausgabeseite immer mehr auseinander klafft. Es bestehen nicht genügend Anreize, Leistungen zwischen den strikt getrennten Sektoren „ambulant" und „stationär" zu verschieben. Die Krankenhäuser sind aus Budgetgründen gezwungen, möglichst alle bisher erbrachten Leistungen zu halten, auch wenn sie schon längst ambulant erbracht werden könnten. Der ambulante Bereich bekommt nicht genügend finanzielle Anreize, um Leistungen aus dem stationären Bereich ambulant erbringen zu wollen.

Ein politisches Ziel der neuen Bundesregierung ist es, die Lohnnebenkosten unter 40% zu drücken. Dazu ist es sicher notwendig, den Beitragssatz in der Krankenversicherung dauerhaft unter 13% zu drücken. Wie sieht die Situation aber tatsächlich aus? Auf der Einnahmenseite werden bis zum Jahr 2001 auf die Krankenversicherungen Belastungen zukommen, die Beitragssatzerhöhungen nach sich ziehen werden. Als Beispiel seien hier die Urteile des Bundesgerichtshofs zu sozialen Abgaben für freiwillig versicherte Rentner und zu Einmalzahlungen genannt sowie die im Zuge der Steuerreform geplante niedrigere Bemessungsgrundlage für Arbeitslose. Auf der Ausgabenseite wird es zu keinen Entlastungen kommen. Der Fortschritt der Medizin und die Verschiebung innerhalb der Alterspyramide der Bevölkerung werden weitere Ausgabensteigerungen nach sich ziehen.

Die konsequente Ausschöpfung von Wirtschaftlichkeitsreserven und der Abbau von vorhandenen Überkapazitäten werden dem Gesundheitssystem so viel Luft verschaffen, dass das System noch ein paar Jahre aufrechterhalten werden kann. Durch eine größere Zielgenauigkeit der Leistungen (dies kann zum Beispiel durch Verordnungsrichtlinien erreicht werden) kann zudem sichergestellt werden, dass die notwendige Leistung im richtigen Rahmen und zum richtigen Preis dem Bedürftigen zukommt.

Riesige Reserven liegen in der Nutzung der neuen Informationstechnologien. Die Zukunft des Gesundheitswesens wird in hohem Maße von neuen Technologien und ihrem verantwortungsvollen Einsatz geprägt sein. Als Beispiel sei die Erweiterung der Chipkarte im Sinne eines Patientenausweises mit medizinischen Daten angeführt. Die Vernetzung der verschiedenen Bereiche des Gesundheitswesens muss schnell und umfassend vorangetrieben werden. Leider versperren viele Barrieren –

vor allem datenschutzrechtlicher Natur – einen sinnvollen Einsatz. Die Initiative D21 wird versuchen ihren Beitrag dazu zu leisten, dass derart restriktive Hemmnisse zum Wohle der versicherten Patienten beseitigt werden können. Die dadurch möglichen Einsparpotentiale liegen auf der Hand; angenommen wir könnten nur 1% unserer Gesamtausgaben einsparen, hätten wir es mit einer Größenordnung von 2,5 Milliarden DM zu tun. Dies ist eine Geldsumme, die so schnell keine Gesundheitsreform an Sparpotenzial realisieren könnte.

Die Einführung von DRG's werden die Krankenhäuser belohnen, die qualitativ gut und wirtschaftlich orientiert arbeiten.

▪ Fazit

▪ Die Einnahmenseite in der gesetzlichen Krankenversicherung wird weiter geschwächt.

▪ Die Ausgabenseite wird trotz Budgetierung weiter wachsen.

▪ Die Erschließung von Wirtschaftlichkeitsreserven durch Rationalisierung und der Abbau von Überkapazitäten können die immer größer werdende Schere zwischen Einnahmen und Ausgaben schließen, zumindest für eine gewisse Zeit.

▪ Innerhalb des nächsten Jahrzehnts wird sich die Gesellschaft die Frage stellen müssen, welche Leistungen aus der Solidargemeinschaft bezahlt werden und welche nicht.

CHAPTER **9** **Socio-ethical remarks on the problem of the distribution of scarce resources in the health system**

H.-P. SCHREIBER

The intention in what follows is to examine the question of the principle underlying the organisation of a fair healthcare provision. In so doing, one needs to start from the general premise that human life generally finds itself in a permanent state of shortage. Nothing is in excess. Everything is scarce; not just external resources, but the resources of our own body also are subject to restrictions. At the same time, however, scarcity makes for invention. And in fact, out of all the inventions which human beings have made in the course of their cultural development to alleviate the distress of scarcity, the institution of social solidarity stands out above all. It constitutes as it were a compensatory system of mutual social care which applies above all to the needy, the weak, the ill and the failures, the unfortunate and the victims. The idea of the interdependent community in its current form is a constituent part of modern societies whose roots date back to the Judaic-Christian characteristics of our Western culture and the associated view of people and the resultant moral concept.

The idea of solidarity attempts to cushion the scarcity of vital resources by a fair redistribution. What does this mean now in terms of the distribution model for medical care? What does a fair health system look like? There are in particular two arguments which counter the frequently advanced contention that healthcare provision should be left solely to the marketplace. In the first place we know that the market has limits. Thus, it is unable to react appropriately, for example, to conditions that threaten the whole community and which incur economic costs to a considerable extent. These include epidemics and dangerous infectious diseases (AIDS) and not least also the phenomenon of deterioration of the general state of health of children in developing countries. To these and similar events the market will never react appropriately. This means that neither the development of medical technology nor the concern about public health can be left to the market alone. Instead society, i.e. the state, must organise healthcare provision collectively in order to ensure a non-means-tested basic medical provision.

Secondly, there is the question of the assessment of the role and value of the 'health' resource, in which we maintain that health is much more than just one subjective need among others. Health, like peace, freedom, safety, even life itself, is a so-called conditional resource. Conditional resources are constituted in such a way that, while they are never everything, without them nothing is possible. Their possession is a precondition for us as humans to achieve our life projects with at least some prospects of success. In times of normality, these resources are unnoticed. As long as we are certain that we possess them, we do not pay them particular attention in everyday life. But as soon as they become scarce, they constitute the sole focus of our concern and our interests. Everything else pales in comparison and the acquisition or re-acquisition of these conditional resources is the sole aim of all our efforts and endeavours.

It is therefore not surprising that the question of how justice is ordained in a society is answered precisely in relation to the importance that a society attributes to these resources: societies which allow a selective shortfall in supply of these resources are not just societies. In view of the numerous gaps in the market in the distribution of such resources, a society that is interested in fairness cannot leave the safeguarding and distribution of such basic social resources to the market. The market knows no fairness, only the purchasing power of the stronger. A social order focussed on justice is characterised specifically by the fact that it guarantees the universal basic provision of these conditional resources to people and hence also the resource of health.

In order to be able to answer the question about a fair method of distribution in the healthcare system, a model should be used in order to attempt to clarify the type of health system that would be admitted by individuals who pursue their own interests under conditions of impartiality. The American social philosopher John Rawls in his theory of justice developed such a model. In this model, people take decisions concealed behind a veil of ignorance with the consequence that they know neither their life expectancy nor their state of health nor their later income nor their future social status. According to Rawls, such people would presumably seek a healthcare system that incorporated both acute treatment and also long-term care, associated with the aim of allowing each of them suitable opportunities to advance their own life in each phase of their individual life. Furthermore, those people acting reasonably behind the veil of ignorance would assume that plans should be laid for a normal life span and that each phase of human life is in principle equal and hence no phase should be neglected simply because it occurred earlier or later. This would then result in healthcare services being apportioned in such a way as to meet the major task over a person's whole life of maintaining or restoring their general ability to live their life. Rawls' model makes it clear that with the idea of the social contract we can develop an argument which provides convincing grounds for an income-neutral, and hence jointly financed, basic care provision.

All this however says nothing yet about the nature and content of the individual claim in respect of the extent of society's obligation and the degree of care provision. What does a fair share of public health care provision available to all cover? We must keep our remarks short. The right to a fair share of public health care provision, as we have already seen, does not allow a maximalist interpretation, because this would go far beyond the concept of fairness. A maximalist health care provision would, among other things, result in the monopolisation of the use of resources by medical progress.

The system that should be promoted out of considerations of fairness is therefore one that ensures general basic medical provision for all. What however should the list of services of basic medical provision contain? What points of view should be highlighted in determining its content?

There is neither a general criterion according to which medical services clearly constitute a constituent of the basic provision, nor do we possess a formal equation for obtaining a basic minimum. In other words, the extent of proper basic medical care provision cannot be definitively determined because this standard is dependent both on the citizens' culturally related level of expectations and also the state of development of medical technology in the country, as well as on the economic capacity of the society. There is therefore no medical algorithm for identifying an obligatory core area of care provision. How can the ethicist make suitable limiting proposals here? The task of ethics in this context can only be to outline a basic framework for a responsible social formulation of the healthcare system in which a basic equality of general provision that is immune to rationing is distinguished from areas of provision that are liable to rationing. Since there is no ethical calculation from which to derive the criteria for an impartial and just care ethic for the rationing of medical resources, nothing else remains for ethics than to refer to the medium of public debate. The exclusion of certain patient groups from certain medical services and the suspension of certain areas of care provision should not be the consequence of a policy of secrecy on the part of the health authorities, etc. That benefit-cost analyses within the health economic field should be embedded in the public debate is already apparent from the vague and semantically open concept of benefit. Nothing is of benefit in itself because beneficial and less beneficial is only ever something in relation to certain interests, values and aims about which, and about the justification and reasonableness of which, one must always be clear when undertaking a solid, benefit-maximising calculation. And in all of this it can be recognised that the area of individual interests, the different concepts of life and the different focuses of quality do not in principle allow a simple operationalisation, as the economy would constantly like to see. Human life has a value and not a price. That is as it were our ethical credo. But it does not follow from this that nothing should be too expensive for health. We will not be able to escape the obligation of rationing in the long term and therefore we must above all also develop quantitative procedures in order to be able to measure the effects of medical services on the quality of life. But the ethics of rationing is still in its infancy. It can be seen today that as a result of the increase in age (demographic factor) and the enormous dynamics of the developments in medical technology in the health care system, as well as in other areas of the welfare state, a welfare-state-based offer-demand mechanism of unrestricted desires and preferences and unrestricted technical possibilities is increasingly overwhelming the capacities of our economy.

In the debates on scarce resources, we must therefore ensure not only economic, but also ethical transparency. In so doing we must above all abandon two illusions: the surplus illusion and the expert illusion. The surplus illusion states that medical provision is sufficiently available; anyone who asks will receive the requested service. The expert illusion states that all decisions relating to allocation can only be justified from the medical side. This thesis ignores the dual aspect of all allocational decisions because, in addition to a medical technology component, these also have an ethical component. For that reason it seems important that ethical decision-making criteria should also increasingly be discussed publicly. The medical practitioner does not have any privileged access to an adequate assessment of the global ethical context on the grounds of his special knowledge. In my opinion this assessment must be reserved for public debate. But just as there is no specific medical jurisdiction over allocational decisions, nor can we leave the allocation of services in the health care system to health bureaucrats and politicians. Transparency in terms of the distribution strategies in the health system is an obligatory requirement of justice in a democratic community. In other words, these strategies must be made public and at the same time gain the approval of the citizens. The increasing requirement for ethical discussions in almost all areas of our modern, welfare-state, industrial and service society is obviously the price we must pay for economic, political, technical and cultural modernisation.

Thus, in the end there remains the concrete question as to how important the population considers a comprehensive insurance against the risk of disease to be, even in old age, and what services it is prepared to provide for this. But this specifically is a question that can only be answered by a public discussion and ultimately by a democratic decision.

■ Sozialethische Anmerkungen zum Problem der Verteilung knapper Güter im Gesundheitswesen

H.-P. Schreiber

Alle menschlichen Gesellschaften sind mit dem Problem konfrontiert, ihren Mitgliedern Güter zuteilen zu müssen. Auch die Natur ist eine Art Verteilungsagentur, jedoch ist ihr Zuteilungsmodus physischer und geistiger Fähigkeiten an den Menschen nicht rechtfertigungspflichtig. Da Verteilungsverfahren in demokratischen Gesellschaften nicht nur begründungs- und zustimmungspflichtig sein müssen, sondern auch gerecht, stellt sich die Frage: Was ist eine gerechte Gesellschaft und insbesondere, was ist ein gerechtes Gesundheitssystem? Drei Modelle bieten sich an: 1. das Modell des reinen Marktes, dem zufolge das Gut der medizinischen Versorgung ausnahmslos privatwirtschaftlich organisiert wird; 2. das Modell des absoluten Wohlfahrtsstaats, in dem die medizinische Versorgung im Rahmen einer umfassenden gesetzlichen Sozialversicherung erfolgt und 3. schließlich das Modell einer Mischung privater und öffentlicher Versorgungsformen. Dieses dritte Modell ist meines Erachtens gegenüber den beiden ersten vorzuziehen, denn bei ihm handelt es sich um ein System, das eine egalitaristisch-marktunabhängige Grundversorgung mit einem differenzierten privaten Versicherungsmarkt kombiniert, und dadurch sowohl dem gleichen Recht eines jeden auf einen fairen Anteil an der öffentlichen Gesundheitsversorgung als auch dem liberalen Prinzip individuell-selbstverantwortlicher Lebensgestaltung und Zukunftsvorsorge ausreichend Rechnung zu tragen vermag.

Die Gerechtigkeitsfrage betrifft jedoch nicht nur die Frage nach dem Versorgungssystem, sondern ebenso auch die Frage nach den Kriterien für eine gerechte Mittelverteilung innerhalb des Leistungsangebotes eines kollektiv organisierten Gesundheitswesens. Bei knappen Mitteln geht es insbesondere um die Ermittlung rationierungsethischer Prinzipien, wobei die Suche danach voraussetzt, dass es Gründe gibt, wichtige von weniger wichtigen Leistungen, zwecknähere von zweckentfernteren Behandlungsmöglichkeiten zu unterscheiden. Da es – wie wir wissen – in der medizinischen Versorgung immer auch Dringlichkeitsgrade gibt, ist jede Rationierungspolitik genötigt, bei der Ermittlung medizinischer Erfolgsparameter medizinische Kompetenz mit ökonomischer Rationalität sowie mit einer gerechtigkeits-ethischen Vernunft zu verbinden.

Rationierung im Gesundheitswesen ist identisch mit der Forderung, jede Form einer maximalistischen Versorgungsregel aufzugeben, derzufolge alles zum gegenwärtigen medizintechnischen Entwicklungsstand

Mögliche allen zukommen zu lassen ist, koste es, was es wolle. Im Weiteren bedeutet Rationierung, dass die Unfinanzierbarkeit eines solchen Versorgungsmaximalismus Knappheiten erzeugt und somit Entscheidungen darüber erforderlich macht, welche Leistungen bzw. Therapien für wen unter welchen Umständen von der kollektiven Versicherung bezahlt werden sollten und welche nicht. Will man ethische Prinzipien für den Umgang mit einem rationierten Leistungsumfang formulieren, dann wird man gleichzeitig auch Kriterien für die Vorzugswürdigkeit bestimmter Leistungen zu ermitteln haben. Und eben dies ist eine ungemein schwierige Aufgabe und es gehört zweifellos zu den strategischen Vorzügen jeder Maximalismusposition, diese Schwierigkeit verschleiern zu können. Wer alles für alle fordert, muss keine Zuteilungsentscheidungen fällen; er kann vorgeben allen wohl zu tun, ohne jemandem weh tun zu müssen. Sobald sich jedoch der Maximalismus als Illusion erweist, wird das Setzen von Prioritäten nötig und es beginnt ein Abwägen des Mehr oder Weniger, ein Vorgang, der Vergleichskriterien erforderlich macht, um Dringlichkeiten bestimmen und Erfolge messen zu können.